NUTRITION FOR RECOVERY

Eating Disorders

NUTRITION FOR RECOVERY

Eating Disorders

Kathryn Reichert, M.S., L.R.D.

Clinical Dietitian
St. Luke's Hospital, Meritcare
Fargo, North Dakota

CRC Press
Boca Raton   Ann Arbor   London   Tokyo

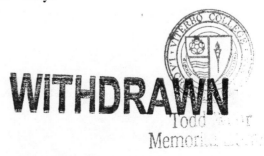

Library of Congress Cataloging-in-Publication Data

Reichert, Kathryn J.
   Nutrition for recovery : eating disorders / author, Kathryn J.
Reichert.
       p.   cm.
   Includes bibliographical references and index.
   ISBN 0-8493-8651-9
   1. Eating disorders—diet therapy.   I. Title.
   [DNLM: 1. Eating Disorders—diet therapy.   2. Nutritional
Requirements.   WM 175 R349n]
   RC552.E18R443   1993
   616.85′260654—dc20
   DNLM/DLC
   for Library of Congress   92-48835
                                                                        CIP

Note: The first section, *A Professional's Guide,* includes worksheets ("Sample Home Meal Plan" and "Your Meal Plan") which may be reproduced by the health care professional for patient use as needed.

NUTRITION FOR RECOVERY: EATING DISORDERS

PREFACE

This work is focused on nutritional therapy for patients with eating disorders. It is most effectively implemented by a registered dietitian as a member of a multidisciplinary team that provides cognitive, behavioral, family, and other therapy approaches.

The first section, *A Professional's Guide,* includes worksheets ("Sample Home Meal Plan" and "Your Meal Plan") which may be reproduced by the health care professional for patient use as needed. (Other pages may not be reproduced in any form, except as noted on the disclaimer page at the front of this book.)

THE AUTHOR

Kathryn Reichert, M.S., L.R.D. is a licensed registered dietitian at St. Luke's Hospitals MeritCare, Fargo, North Dakota. Her specialty areas include geriatric nutrition, renal nutrition, and nutrition for eating-disordered patients. Ms. Reichert was the dietitian for St. Luke's Hospitals MeritCare Inpatient Eating Disorders Program from 1987 to 1989.

Ms. Reichert graduated in 1974 from The College of St. Catherine, St. Paul, Minnesota with a B.A. degree in Foods and Nutrition. She obtained an M.S. degree in Nutrition at Case Western Reserve University, Cleveland, Ohio in 1975.

Ms. Reichert is a member of The American Dietetic Association and the North Dakota Dietetic Association.

Ms. Reichert has presented lectures to the public and health professionals on the topics of geriatric nutrition and nutrition for eating disorders.

ACKNOWLEDGMENTS

I wish to acknowledge the expertise of Dr. David Abbott and other MeritCare Eating Disorders Program Staff who integrated the concepts of the three-dimensional model and the learning curve into the inpatient program design.

In addition, I would like to thank the following people for their review and suggestions:

Debra Nelson, R.N., B.S.N., Coordinator, MeritCare Eating Disorders Program

Linda Schander, L.R.D., MeritCare Eating Disorders Program

Stephen Wonderlich, Ph.D., Co-Director, MeritCare Eating Disorders Program; Associate Professor, Department of Psychiatry, University of North Dakota, School of Medicine

Further, I wish to acknowledge the important feedback and suggestions offered by patients of the MeritCare Inpatient Eating Disorders Program, St. Luke's Hospitals MeritCare, Fargo, North Dakota.

I appreciate the assistance given by many restaurant and food companies in providing nutrition information about their products.

PROFESSIONAL'S GUIDE

YOUR HOME MEAL PLAN

CLASS OUTLINES

PROFESSIONAL'S GUIDE

ACKNOWLEDGMENTS

I wish to thank the following people for their review and suggestions:

David Abbott, M.D., Co-Director, MeritCare Eating Disorders Program/Director, St. Luke's Hospitals MeritCare Inpatient Eating Disorders Program

Debra Nelson, R.N., B.S.N., Coordinator, MeritCare Eating Disorders Program

Linda Schander, L.R.D., MeritCare Eating Disorders Program

Stephen Wonderlich, Ph.D., Co-Director, MeritCare Eating Disorders Program; Associate Professor, Department of Psychiatry, University of North Dakota, School of Medicine

I. INTRODUCTION

Nutrition For Recovery: Eating Disorders has been based upon concepts presented in St. Luke's Hospitals/Fargo Clinic Inpatient/Outpatient Eating Disorders Programs. Therefore, the nutrition education components — meal planning system and class outlines — are developed for use in both inpatient and outpatient settings.

The following will identify both similarities and differences existing between inpatient and outpatient treatment settings.

A. Similarities: Inpatient and Outpatient Treatment

1. Program Goals — Broad Approaches

Broad program goals include restoration of health and relapse prevention. Relapse prevention is a self-control program aimed at maintaining recovery. The basis of relapse prevention is to teach the patient key coping strategies with skill-building methods. Coping strategies include effective problem-solving techniques, assertiveness skills, positive self-dialogue skills, stress management and meal planning. Skill-training methods involve instruction, modeling and behavioral rehearsal. The patient can expect gradual ease in using these skills and greater effectiveness in their use as the skills become better established. A recommended text on this subject is *Relapse Prevention: Maintenance Strategies in the Treatment of Addiction* by J. Gordon and G. A. Marlatt, editors.[1]

Another element utilized in both programs is the cognitive-behavioral approach to treatment. With this approach, it is recognized that dysfunctional beliefs concerning weight and body image are key in perpetuating eating disorders. Treatment is then focused upon identifying and assessing dysfunctional thoughts, feelings and behavior regarding their usefulness in achieving goals. Alternative thinking and behavioral patterns (coping strategies) are developed and practiced by the patient to replace former dysfunctional beliefs and unhealthy behavior.

2. Nutritional Assessment

In these programs, anthropometric measurements including mid-arm circumference, triceps skinfold and mid-arm muscle circumference have not been routinely done. The rationale: for underweight patients, both lean body mass and fat tissue reserves will be restored given a healthy distribution of carbohydrate, protein and fat in meal plans, adequate levels of exercise and appropriate rates of weight gain in the programs, if indicated.

Chemistries of interest include but are not limited to hemoglobin, hematocrit, albumin, sodium, potassium, magnesium, phosphorus and chloride. Somatomdein-C, nitrogen balance, 24 hour urinary creatinine and oxygen consumption studies have not been routinely conducted for reasons cited in the paragraph above and to help moderate costs of treatment.

A supplemental multivitamin with minerals at 100% of the RDA is provided to patients until healthy eating has been sustained in order to hasten repletion of possible marginal nutrient reserves such as zinc, iron and B vitamins. After healthy eating is established, patients are advised that supplementation can be discontinued because the home meal plan will cover nutritional needs.

3. Dietitian's Role/Nutrition Education

In addition to developing individualized home meal plans for patients, the dietitian provides group nutrition classes as a framework to challenge common misconceptions and to explain the rationale for the meal planning system. Topics included in *Nutrition For Recovery: Eating Disorders* class outlines include guidelines for healthy eating, the body's use of energy sources, set point theory, adverse effects of dieting, calcium nutrition and relapse prevention.

Complementary activities to reinforce class content may be added such as clipping magazine/newspaper photographs of ultra-thin models, identifying food models with food groups, estimating actual food portions and viewing educational videotapes. A recommended videotape, *The Waist Land: Why Diets Don't Work* can be used as an introduction to the class "The Dieting Addiciton". Ordering information for this videotape is shown on the Reference section.[2] Replica food models are a useful means to estimate food portions; ordering information is also included in the Reference section.[3]

In addition to structured classes, group question and answer sessions have allowed patients to bring forth additional nutrition topics of interest. The annotated bibliography includes information that can be cited in response to questions frequently asked in these sessions.

Because of the complexity of meal planning and the need to address multiple nutrition misconceptions held by the patient, it is recommended that this system be used by a registered dietitian. In addition, this system will require modification if other medical concerns exist, for example: diabetes mellitus, chronic lactose intolerance, food allergies, use of MAOI antidepressants, or resumption of athletic activities (if not in conflict with recovery).

B. Inpatient Program Structure

A multidisciplinary team approach has been used in the inpatient program. Core staff members include the psychiatrist, primary nurse, occupational therapist, dietitian and social worker. Additional team members may include a psychologist, medical specialist, chemical dependency counselor, tutor and mental health care professionals previously involved in the patient's care. A coordinated treatment plan is achieved through weekly team conferences in which treatment goals and methods are defined. In addition, daily informal updates by core team members review patient progress and the need for any modification to goals established for the week. Adequate communication among staff is essential for a consistent team approach to the patient. This, in turn, facilitates patient trust and builds the "therapeutic alliance" between the patient and the team.

The inpatient program has been divided into five phases. Each phase has defined goals to be met before a patient progresses to the next phase. The first two phases are highly structured with limited decision making by the patient. This results in rapid patient compliance to the program protocol and minimizes entanglement with frequently observed cognitive impairment of patients such as decreased concentration, memory and motivation. (These impairments, if present, become less pronounced following refeeding and for some patients, anti-depressant therapy.) The last three program phases shift to increased decision making by the patient. By the fifth phase, the patient is determining his/her own treatment objectives by applying coping strategies learned in previous phases to self-identified high-risk situations. In this phase, the team encourages independence in a supportive role by assisting the patient in evaluating coping strategies used in response to specific risk exposures. Throughout the program, a combination of individual, group and family therapy is used. By these means, broad program goals — restoration of health and relapse prevention — are addressed.

C. Refeeding Progression for Inpatient Program

Upon hospital admission, all patients are prescribed a nonselective 1200 calorie meal plan with features that minimize possible refeeding problems. Features include 3 grams of sodium, low lactose, low fat and 6 feedings. After approximately 7 to 10 days of refeeding, these features are discontinued in most cases. Nonselective meals and snacks are continued through the first three program phases. Specific food preferences and aversions are not accommodated with the exception of medically documented food allergies or religious-based restrictions. Throughout the third phase, one high-risk food per day is chosen by the dietitian from a specific list of high-risk foods previously identified by the patient and is sent to the patient. (The high-risk food is substituted in place of calorically equivalent menu or snack foods.) Repeated exposure to high-risk foods is intended to decrease patients' apprehension to those foods.

The calorie level is adjusted per tri-weekly documented patient weights until the midpoint of the recommended weight range is achieved. The desired rate of weight gain for severely underweight anorectic patients is 3 pounds per week. To accomplish this, the calorie level is usually progressed by 300 calorie increments which can often result in a peak intake of up to 4800 calories or more per day. For bulimic patients who do not require weight restoration, the calorie level is progressed by 300 calorie increments to usual levels of 1500 or 1800 calories per day for weight stabilization. Weight status is not shared with the patient until the midpoint of the recommended weight range is reached. Patients are then informed of the recommended weight range and are allowed to observe one weight check each week for the remainder of hospitalization.

When the patient has attained sufficient weight and other criteria of the third phase have been met, the patient is advanced to the fourth phase. At this time the dietitian and patient compare previous unhealthy eating behaviors with anticipated healthy food choices and meal/snack schedule following hospitalization. A weight maintenance home meal plan is developed based upon these predictions. In the fourth and fifth program phases, the patient selects meal and snack items from the regular hospital menu and snack inventory according to the home meal plan. Meal and snack choices are checked closely by the dietitian at menu planning sessions to ensure that the patient is selecting a variety of foods in adequate amounts. Menu planning sessions provide the opportunity to review pertinent concepts if/when the patient is reluctant to choose up to the plan. As the patient gains confidence in using the home meal plan, he/she is asked to identify high-risk situations that may involve food. Common examples include: grocery shopping, eating out, cooking, going through the hospital cafeteria to select and eat a meal and eating with family members at home. These situations, as well as other non food-related situations are rehearsed in the fifth phase as previously mentioned.

Various team members confer with the patient's family, as needed, to advise them of supportive interaction. If the patient plans to live with other family members after hospital discharge, the dietitian highlights meal planning concepts in a joint conference with the patient and family. Ideas discussed include the patient's responsibility to plan food intake, shared communication regarding grocery shopping, expanded food choices to avoid former patterns of separate cooking for the patient versus family, and patient autonomy in food-related issues.

D. Trends in Inpatient Programming

Length of stay is becoming abbreviated for two primary reasons: declining inpatient insurance coverage and more effective outpatient treatment. In the original program, a typical length of stay for a bulimic patient was three to four weeks. In order for an anorectic patient to achieve weight restoration up to the recommended weight range, generally eight to 12 weeks of hospitalization was required. It is projected that length of hospitalization may become limited to three to five days for a bulimic patient and seven to 14 days for an anorectic patient. In this reduced time frame, goals will include fluid and electrolyte stabilization, facilitating the patient's efforts to begin normalized eating and home meal plan instruction. Thus, hospitalization for the treatment of eating disorders is becoming focused on crisis intervention. The majority of cognitive-behavioral therapy (and weight restoration, if indicated) is taking place in the outpatient setting. Another option is day hospitalization which can serve as a transition between full hospitalization and outpatient treatment.

E. Outpatient Program

Multidisciplinary team members include the psychiatrist, nurse specialist and dietitian. Group classes and individual counseling are provided for patients with bulimia nervosa. Individual counseling is the primary treatment approach used for patients with anorexia nervosa.

Expected rate of weight gain and calorie increments used for anorectic patients differ from the inpatient to the outpatient setting. Weight gains of 1/4 to 1/2 pound per week are realistic in outpatient treatment. It is recommended that the initial calorie level be set at no more than 300 calories above pretreatment intake levels in order to secure patient compliance. Calorie increments of 150 to 250 calories to the specific meal plan per week for weight gain are appropriate. In contrast to inpatient treatment, weight restoration in the outpatient setting runs a lengthy course with the possibility of setbacks along the way.

II. ESTABLISHING A RECOMMENDED WEIGHT RANGE

Before developing a weight maintenance meal plan in either an inpatient or outpatient program, a recommended weight range needs to be determined. It is appropriate to set a range rather than a single number in order to allow for normal weight fluctuations. Such fluctuations are caused by many factors such as the menstrual cycle, temporary water retention following intake of high sodium foods, amount of food or beverage recently consumed, accuracy of the scale being used, time of day weight is measured and weight of clothing. A 5-pound weight range has frequently been used in the program. For patients who have experienced significant weight gain as a consequence of bulimia, the weight range may be stated as the current weight or lower.

Several methods may be considered in arriving at a recommended weight range. Methods described in the following section are used for both adolescent and adult patients. However, for any female patient, age 16 or younger (or male patient, age 18 or younger), the recommended weight range can best be stated as a short-term range. Age-related growth can justify an upward adjustment to a recommended weight range.

A. Anorexia Nervosa

The professional may wish to set a weight range with the midpoint at the lowest number given for a stated height from average body weight tables such as the 1959 Metropolitan Life Insurance Tables (Table 1 in Appendix). Another option to the above methods is to establish a range beginning at 90% of the calculations shown below. (This is the preferred method in our programs.)

Female Patient — 100 pounds for the first 5 feet + 5 pounds for each additional inch.

Male Patient — 106 pounds for the first 5 feet + 6 pounds for each additional inch.

Example: female anorectic patient, age 16 years, height 5 feet 6 inches.

5 feet	100 pounds
6 inches × 5 pounds per inch	+ 30 pounds
	130 pounds

130 pounds × 90% = 117 pounds
Recommended weight range: 117-122 pounds
(Begin the 5-pound range at 90% of the calculations.)

To strengthen the decision of weight range, other aspects can be evaluated. Reference can be made to the nomograms developed by Frish and McArthur (Table 2 in Appendix) for minimal weight required for onset or resumption of menses.[5]

A patient's goal weight range may be adjusted if the patient's history suggests that at full mature height, regular menstrual cycles occurred at a lower weight. To illustrate this with the example shown above, a 16-year-old patient had maintained regular menstrual cycles at a predisorder weight of 114 pounds. The professional may wish to set the goal weight range at 114 to 119 pounds.

If the anorectic patient is not substantially underweight, the goal may be to stabilize current weight stated as a range.

B. Bulimia Nervosa

For the bulimic adolescent or adult without need for weight restoration, emphasis is placed on normalized eating and weight stabilization. If current weight is similar to predisorder weight, an important patient goal will be the acceptance of current weight. It is essential for the patient to resist the desire to attain a lower weight goal.

If significant weight gain has occurred since the onset of the disorder and is above average weight-for-height tables, it is recommended to refrain from setting a lower weight range. It is more appropriate to persuade the patient away from any direct intent of weight loss since this is an addictive force of bulimia. Instead, emphasizing the priority of normalizing eating behaviors for the goal of weight stabilization and avoiding further weight gain is more appropriate. In fact, normalized eating may allow the body to reset its set point — without chronic dieting — toward usual body weight.

Example: Female bulimic patient, age 30, height 64 inches, current weight 135 pounds. Predisorder weight history: stable between 118 to 125 pounds. Patient's stated weight goal: 100 pounds. Recommended weight range: current weight or lower. (When calculating daily calorie requirements in the following section, actual weight of 135 pounds would be used.)

III. DEVELOPING A MEAL PLAN

After the recommended weight range has been established, a prediction can be calculated for a weight maintenance calorie level. From this estimate of daily calorie requirement, the dietitian can calculate desirable intake in grams of total carbohydrate, protein and fat. The final step involves determining appropriate number of food units from each core food group which will provide a desirable proportion of carbohydrate, protein and fat. An explanation of calculations and examples are as follows.

A. Estimating Weight Maintenance Calorie Requirements

1. Anorexia Nervosa

After the recovering anorectic patient has completed weight restoration, the Harris-Benedict method of estimating baseline resting energy requirements (REE) can be used. The REE is then multiplied by an adjustment factor (AF) to derive the estimated total daily energy requirement.

REE × AF = maintenance calorie level
REE for women: 655 + [(9.6 × weight in kg) + (1.7 × height in cm) - (4.7 × age in years)]
REE for men: 66 + [(13.7 × weight in kg) + (5 × height in cm) - (6.8 × age in years)]
Conversion factors: 2.2 pounds = 1 kg
1 inch = 2.54 cm

The metabolic states of most patients who have achieved significant weight restoration require a higher adjustment factor than a commonly used factor of 1.25. From our experience, an increased adjustment factor of 1.8 is recommended.

REE × 1.8 = maintenance calorie level for a weight-restored anorectic patient.

Example: female anorectic patient, age 16, height 5 feet 6 inches. Recommended weight range: 117 to 122 pounds. Midpoint of recommended weight range: 119.5 pounds.

Conversions: 119.5 pounds ÷ 2.2 pounds per kg = 54 kg
5 feet 6 inches × 2.54 cm per inch = 168 cm
REE = 655 + (9.6 x 54) + (1.7 × 168) – (4.7 × 16)
REE = 1384 calories
1384 calories × 1.8 = 2491 calories estimated for weight maintenance.
(2500 calories will be used in calculations to follow.)

2. Bulimia Nervosa

These patients frequently present with weights at or somewhat above their usual healthy body weight history or average body weight-for-height tables. If a patient's current weight occurs above these points of reference, a low calorie, weight reduction meal plan is avoided since this is a strong set up for relapse. An intentional weight loss program also sends the wrong message to the patient by reinforcing his/her fear of "feeling fat." The goal is to set a calorie level for these patients that will stabilize current weight while providing sufficient amounts of food to reasonably satisfy the appetite.

For bulimic patients, the same equation for calculating REE can be used. However, initial energy needs for weight maintenance may be lower than the usual adjustment factor of 1.25. Therefore, an initial adjustment factor of 1.15 is suggested.

Example: Female bulimic patient, age 30, height 64 inches. Current weight: 135 pounds. Recommended weight range: current weight or lower.

Conversion: 135 pounds ÷ 2.2 pounds per kg = 61 kg
64 inches × 2.54 cm per inch = 163 cm
REE = 655 + (9.6 x 61) + (1.7 x 163) - (4.7 × 30)
REE = 1377 calories
1377 calories × 1.15 = 1584 calories for weight maintenance.
(1600 calories will be used in calculations to follow.)

B. Desirable Intake of Carbohydrate, Protein, and Fat in Grams

1. Current recommendations for healthy eating suggest that of daily caloric intake, approximately:

   50 to 58% of calories be derived from carbohydrate,
   12 to 20% of calories be derived from protein, and
   30% or fewer calories be derived from fat.

2. To convert calories to grams of carbohydrate, protein and fat, use these conversion factors:

   1 gram of carbohydrate yields 4 calories,
   1 gram of protein yields 4 calories, and
   1 gram of fat yields 9 calories.

3. General Considerations

   (a) According to the 1989 Recommended Dietary Allowances, daily protein intake should generally meet or exceed these levels:[6]

Females from age 11 through 24	46 g or more
Females from age 25 and older	50 g or more
Pregnant females	60 g or more
Lactating females	65 g or more
Males from age 11 through 14	58 g or more
Males from age 15 through 24	59 g or more
Males from age 25 and older	63 g or more

   (b) For intakes of greater than 2000 calories per day, it may be advantageous to select a higher percentage of carbohydrate intake (55 to 58% of total calories), select a middle percentage of protein intake (15 to 18% of total calories) and choose a lower percentage of fat intake (25 to 27% of total calories). These percentages will moderate intake of the complete protein and fat food groups that are often more challenging for the anorectic patient to consume. For intakes of 2000 calories or less, selecting percentages at or close to 50% of calories as carbohydrate, 20% of calories as protein and 30% of calories as fat usually results in a feasible division of food groups.

C. Distributing Total Grams of Carbohydrate, Protein, and Fat Into Core Food Groups

1. The American Diabetes/Dietetic's Associations (ADA) exchange lists are used as a basis for this system's core food groups.[7] Nomenclature of the exchange lists and of this system is included. Each core food group is given a standard amount of carbohydrate, protein and fat per unit as shown.

   Table 3 (See Appendix). ADA Exchange Lists and Core Food Groups:

   For the eating disorders programs, terminology of some food groups have been altered due to negative connotations frequently associated with the words meat and fat. The terms "complete protein" and "complement" have been used respectively. However, to simplify use of *Nutrition For Recovery: Eating Disorders* by health professionals, food group titles conform more closely to familiar terminology of the American Diabetes/Dietetics Associations.

Table 4 (See Appendix):

A comparison of the Canadian Diabetes Association's Choice System and core food groups from *Nutrition For Recovery: Eating Disorders* is shown in the Appendix to facilitate use of this program by Canadian health professionals.[8]

2. Additional Considerations

   a. Limit the number of complete protein units recommended up to seven units per day for the purpose of moderating cholesterol intake. For this food group, a range of units may be stated such as five to seven units. This flexibility may allow the patient to feel more at ease when visually estimating portions of meat.

   b. Limit vegetables up to three units per day since excessive intake of these foods may decrease intake of foods from other groups.

   c. For most patients, grain and fruit units may be similar in number or grains may somewhat exceed fruit units.

   d. Encourage all patients to include at least two units from the milk group per day. Three units from the milk group daily will ensure adequate calcium intake for this population at high risk of developing osteoporosis. Frequent consumption of other high calcium foods is encouraged. This is particularly important for those patients who dislike consuming fluid milk and yogurt. Two versions of the milk group are provided in the meal planning system. Select the appropriate page for your patient depending upon if he/she consumes skim milk or 2% milk at home.

   e. If the patient indicates that he/she intends to consume only one or less units from the milk group daily, it may be advantageous to select a lower percentage for protein. Conversely, if a patient opts to consume three or more units per day from the milk group, using a higher percentage of protein (17 to 20%) may be appropriate.

   f. If a patient is reluctant to use margarine or other fat units on bread or toast, it may be advisable to select a lower percentage of fat (20 to 25% of total calories). In this situation, the patient may be able to use the lesser number of fat units when melted over other grain units and vegetables. Patients may prefer to drink 2% or whole milk instead of skim milk when told that use of 2% of whole milk will reduce the number of fat units recommended on the meal plan.

   g. If the patient anticipates that he/she will be routinely eating snacks, it will be important to be aware of typical snack choices. These choices can further influence the division of calories into carbohydrate, protein and fat.

   h. If the patient is participating in a school lunch program, it is helpful to relate this program to the meal planning system. The following guidelines may be helpful in discussing the school lunch program.

      (1) In order for the school to receive federal reimbursement, a student must take a minimum of three foods.

      (2) In most schools, 8-ounce cartons of skim, 2% and whole milk are available.

      (3) The average portion of meat served is 2 ounces, cooked weight.

(4) Each menu must offer a total of 3/4 cup fruit and/or vegetable. Combinations may include two fruit servings, two vegetable servings or one fruit and one vegetable serving.

(5) Each menu must offer a total of two servings of bread, rice or pasta.

(6) Bread and buns are usually served without added fat. Vegetables may be served with or without added fat.

(7) School lunch menus are available in advance which facilitates meal planning efforts. Menus are often printed in the local newspapers, posted in schools and included in school newsletters.

(8) If the menu is offering an entree which is a high-risk food or a disliked food, the student may opt to bring a sack lunch from home.

D. Example: 2500 calorie home meal plan calculations for an anorectic patient.

Considerations:

- The patient anticipates drinking 3 cups of skim milk daily.

- The patient is willing to use margarine on grains and vegetables.

- The patient plans to eat two snacks each day; frequent choices are likely to be cheese, crackers, fruit and cookies.

- The patient will participate in the school lunch program; skim milk is available.

1. Section III-B in outline: desirable intake of carbohydrate, protein and fat in grams.

carbohydrate	$56\% \times 2500 = 1400$ calories derived from carbohydrate
	1400 calories ÷ 4 calories per gram = 350 grams carbohydrate
protein	$17\% \times 2500 = 425$ calories derived from protein
	425 calories ÷ 4 calories per gram = 106 grams protein
fat	$27\% \times 2500 = 675$ calories derived from fat
	675 calories ÷ 9 calories per gram = 75 grams fat

2. Section III-C in outline: distributing total grams of carbohydrate, protein and fat into core food groups.

   a. Divide 350 grams of carbohydrate among food groups.

      (1) 3 cups of skim milk provide 36 grams of carbohydrate (and 24 grams of protein).

      (2) Three vegetable units provide 15 grams of carbohydrate (and 6 grams of protein).

      (3) The remaining carbohydrate (299 grams) can be distributed equally between grain and fruit groups. 299 grams ÷ 15 grams per unit of grain or fruit = 20 total units such as 10 grain and 10 fruit units. 10 units of grain will also provide 30 grams of protein.

   b. Divide 106 grams of protein among food groups.

      (1) The milk, vegetable and grain groups planned supply a total of 60 grams of protein.

(2) The remaining protein (46 grams) can be assigned to the complete protein group. 46 grams ÷ 7 grams per unit of complete protein = 6.5 units. In the home meal plan, this can be indicated as 6-7 complete protein units. 6.5 units will provide approximately 32.5 grams of fat.

c. Divide 75 grams of fat among food groups. All food units listed above supply a total of 32.5 grams of fat. The remaining fat (42.5 grams) will be assigned to the fat group. 42.5 grams ÷ 5 grams of fat per fat unit = 8.5 fat units. This may be stated as 8-9 fat units in the home meal plan.

E. Example: 1600 calorie home meal plan calculations for a bulimic patient.

Considerations:

- The patient will consume 1 1/2 cups of skim milk per day.
- The patient will eat one to two units of vegetable daily.
- The patient is accustomed to using margarine and other fat units on a variety of foods.
- The patient dislikes canned fruit; availability of fresh fruit at home is limited.
- The patient anticipates including an evening snack consisting of low-risk food options such as milk, fruit or a sandwich.

1. Section III-B in outline: desirable intake of carbohydrate, protein and fat in grams.

carbohydrate 50% × 1600 = 800 calories derived from carbohydrate
800 calories ÷ 4 calories per gram = 200 grams of carbohydrate
protein 20% × 1600 = 320 calories derived from protein
320 calories ÷ 4 calories per gram = 80 grams of protein
fat 30% × 1600 = 480 calories derived from fat
480 calories ÷ 9 calories per gram = 53 grams of fat

2. Section III-C in outline: distributing total grams of carbohydrate, protein and fat into core food groups.

a. Divide 200 grams of carbohydrate among food groups.

(1) 1 1/2 cups of skim milk provide 18 grams of carbohydrate (and 12 grams of protein).

(2) An average of 1.5 vegetable units per day provide approximately 8 grams of carbohydrate (and 3 grams of protein).

(3) The remaining carbohydrate (174 grams) can be distributed between grain and fruit groups. When considering availability and patient preferences for fruit, more of the remaining carbohydrate can be derived form the grain group such as eight grain units and four fruit groups. Eight units of grain will also supply 24 grams of protein.

b. Divide 80 grams of protein among food groups.

(1) The units planned above provide 39 grams of protein.

(2) The remaining protein (41 grams) will be derived from the complete

protein group. 41 grams # 7 grams per unit of complete protein = approximately six complete protein units. This could be indicated as five to seven complete protein units on the home meal plan. Six complete protein units will provide 30 grams of fat.

   c. Divide 53 grams of fat among food groups. All food units listed above provide a total of 30 grams of fat. The remaining fat (23 grams) will be assigned to the fat group. 23 grams # 5 grams of fat per fat unit = approximately five fat units.

4. Sample meal plan sheets and menus based on the two weight maintenance meal plans are shown later in this section.

IV. MONITORING THE MEAL PLAN

A. Weight Deviations

Any method used in estimating weight maintenance energy needs is imperfect and may result in the need to adjust the home meal plan. For any individual, chronic dieting may or may not impair the body's ability to resume normal metabolic rate which accounts for approximately 70% of total energy needs for most people. If a change in metabolic rate occurs in response to normalized eating, the period of adaptation is open to question. Also, the impact of laxative or diet pill abuse may further impair the accuracy of predicting energy requirements. Therefore, ongoing weekly or bi-monthly weight checks done by a follow-up health professional is recommended. Should problems occur with meal plan compliance or if a patient's weight consistently falls out of the recommended weight range, consultation with a dietitian is warranted. Occasional minor weight deviations from the weight range may be dismissed on the basis of day-to-day variables not associated with an eating disorder.

B. Increased Appetite: Bulimia Nervosa

If a patient with a history of bulimia reports strong hunger drives (other than normal hunger experienced shortly before meals) or a significant rate of weight loss occurs (greater than 1 pound per week) the calorie level may warrant an increase. Because hunger is a strong trigger for binging, the dietitian needs to question the patient regarding the existence of unsettling hunger while following the home meal plan. If this is the case, moderately increasing the plan by 200 to 300 calories, reviewing the importance of eating meals at well-spaced intervals and discussing healthy exercise habits may resolve this problem.

C. Exercise

Usual guidelines for exercise given to patients are 20 to 30 minutes of aerobic exercise three to five times per week above general daily life activities. This level of exercise is consistent with maintaining cardiovascular fitness and serves as a regulator of appetite. Levels of exercise significantly above this recommendation merit the question: Is the patient undertaking exercise for the inappropriate goal of losing weight? If the motive is independent of the eating disorder, calories to meet increased energy needs can be estimated from tables found in various sports nutrition references. Examples include the American Dietetic Association's text, *Sports Nutrition — A Guide for the Professional Working with Active People,* and Katch and McArdle's *Nutrition, Weight Control and Exercise.*[9, 10] Examples of legitimate reasons for high activity levels are resuming participation in a predisorder sport, occupation or continuing with an athletic scholarship program.

D. Inclusion of Food Groups

Patients may request an alteration of how foods are divided among food groups. To increase likelihood of compliance to the meal plan, it is advisable to respond to these requests within the framework of heathy eating. On occasion this may not be fully accommodated. For example, it is suggested that all core food groups be represented in the plan. Also, total avoidance of meats is not advised unless the patient is vegetarian due to religious beliefs. If one or more core food groups is especially troublesome, it may be helpful for the patient to list a food hierarchy ranking low-risk foods to high-risk foods. A patient can then be encouraged to repeatedly try one risk food at a time starting with low-risk foods.

E. Follow-up

A percentage of patients may live a significant distance from the eating disorders treatment center and therefore will not return for follow-up care. Discharge planning includes the coordination of follow-up care for these patients. After obtaining written patient consent, a psychiatrist or mental health counselor and dietitian are contacted at a facility convenient to the patient. In the inpatient program, the dietitian has relayed specific recommendations to the follow-up dietitian by means of a telephone conference. The patient is advised to bring his/her meal planning materials to the initial appointment with the follow-up dietitian.

Appendix

Table 1
1959 Metropolitan Life Insurance Height/Weight Tables

Height without shoes		Weight in pounds without clothing (women)	Weight in pounds without clothing (men)
Feet	Inches		
4	9	90–118	
4	10	92–121	
4	11	95–124	
5	0	98–127	
5	1	101–130	105–134
5	2	104–134	108–137
5	3	107–138	111–141
5	4	110–142	114–145
5	5	114–146	117–149
5	6	118–150	121–154
5	7	122–154	125–159
5	8	126–159	129–163
5	9	130–164	133–167
5	10	134–169	137–172
5	11	141–177	
6	0	145–182	
6	1	149–187	
6	3	157–197	

Adapted from "Statistical Bulletin," Vol. 64, No 1, pp. 6-7. Metropolitan Life Insurance Company. Printed with permission.

Table 2.
Minimum Weight for Height Necessary for
Menstrual Cycles

Height (inches)	(cm)	Menarche or primary amenorrhea			Secondary amenorrhea		
		Min. weight[a] (10th percentile)		Av. weight (50th percentile)	Min. weight[b] (10th percentile)		Av. weight (50th percentile)
		(lb.)	(kg)	(kg)	(lb.)	(kg)	(kg)
53.1	135	66.7	30.3	34.9	74.6	33.9	38.9
53.9	137	68.6	31.2	36.0	76.8	34.9	40.1
54.7	139	70.6	32.1	37.0	79.0	35.9	41.2
55.5	141	72.6	33.0	38.0	81.2	36.9	42.4
56.3	143	74.4	33.8	39.0	83.4	37.9	43.5
57.1	145	76.3	34.7	40.1	85.6	38.9	44.7
57.9	147	78.3	35.6	41.1	87.8	39.9	45.8
58.7	149	80.3	36.5	42.1	90.0	40.9	47.0
59.4	151	82.3	37.4	43.1	92.2	41.9	48.1
60.2	153	84.3	38.3	44.2	94.4	42.9	49.3
61.0	155	86.2	39.2	45.2	96.6	43.9	50.4
61.8	157	88.2	40.1	46.2	98.8	44.9	51.5
62.6	159	90.2	41.0	47.2	101.0	45.9	52.7
63.4	161	92.2	41.9	48.3	103.2	46.9	53.8
64.2	163	93.9	42.7	49.3	105.4	47.9	55.0
65.0	165	95.9	43.6	50.3	107.6	48.9	56.1
65.7	167	97.9	44.5	51.4	109.8	49.9	57.3
66.5	169	99.9	45.4	52.4	112.0	50.9	58.4
67.3	171	101.9	46.3	53.4	114.0	51.8	59.6
68.1	173	103.8	47.2	54.4	116.2	52.8	60.7
68.9	175	105.8	48.1	55.5	118.4	53.8	61.8
69.7	177	107.8	49.0	56.5	120.6	54.8	63.0
70.5	179	109.6	49.8	57.5	112.8	55.8	64.1
71.3	181	111.8	50.8	58.5	125.2	56.9	65.3

[a] Equivalent to 17% fat/body weight. Height growth must be completed or nearing completion.
[b] Equivalent to 22% fat/body weight.

Minimal weight for height necessary for the onset or restoration of menstrual cycles as shown on the 10th percentile. Standards apply to women of ages 16 years and older of Caucasian American or European descent.

From "Menstrual Cycles: Fatness as a Determinant of Minimum Weight for Height Necessary for their Maintenance or Onset" by R.E. Frisch and J.W. McArthur, 1974, *Science*, 185, 949-951. Copyright 1974 by the American Association for the Advancement of Science. Reprinted by permission of the publisher and authors.

Table 3.
ADA Exchange Lists and Core Food Groups

ADA exchange lists	Core food group	Carbohydrate (grams)	Protein (grams)	Fat (grams)
Meat	Complete Protein (subgroup 2)	—	7	5
Fat	Fat	—	—	5
Bread	Grain	15	3	—
Vegetables	Vegetables	5	2	—
Fruit	Fruit	15	—	—
Milk, Skim	Milk, Skim	12	8	—
Milk, 2%	Milk, 2%	12	8	5
Milk, Whole	Milk, Whole	12	8	8

Adapted from *Exchange Lists For Meal Planning*, a meal planning system designed by a committee of the American Diabetes Association and the American Dietetic Association. (While primarily designed for people with diabetes and others who must follow special diets, the exchange lists are based on principles of good nutrition that apply to everyone.) © 1989 American Diabetes Association, The American Dietetic Association. Printed with permission.

Table 4.
Comparison of *Nutrition For Recovery: Eating Disorders* and Canadian Food Group Systems

Nutrition For Recovery: Eating Disorders Core Food Groups		Canadian Diabetes Association Choice System
1 Complete Protein — Subgroup 1	=	1 Protein Foods
1 Complete Protein — Subgroup 2	=	1 Protein + 1/2 Fats and Oils
1 Complete Protein — Subgroup 3	=	1 Protein + 1 Fats and Oils
1 Fat	=	1 Fats and Oils
1 Grain	=	1 Starchy Foods
1 Vegetable	=	1/2 Fruits and Vegetables
(no similar group)	=	Extra Vegetables
1 Fruit	=	1 1/2 Fruits and Vegetables
1 Milk (Skim)	=	2 Milk (Skim)

Reproducible Worksheets

YOUR MEAL PLAN

Name_____   Date_____

Daily Meal Plan Units

_____Complete Protein

_____Fat

_____Grain

_____Vegetable

_____Fruit

_____Milk (Skim)

Sample Distribution of Units in Meals and Snacks

MEALS	SNACKS
_____Complete Protein	_____Complete Protein
_____Fat	_____Fat
_____Grain	_____Grain
_____Vegetable	_____Vegetable
_____Fruit	_____Fruit
_____Milk	_____Milk

SAMPLE HOME MEAL PLAN[11]

FOOD ITEM	FOOD GROUP							
	AMOUNT	COMPLETE PROTEIN	FAT	GRAIN	VEGIES	FRUITS	MILK	CUPS OF FLUID
TIME								
B R E A K F A S T								
TIME								
L U N C H								
TIME								
S U P P E R								
S N A C K S								
TOTAL NUMBER OF FOOD UNITS								

YOUR MEAL PLAN

Name _MAINTENANCE MEAL PLAN_   Date_____
   (ANOREXIA NERVOSA)

Daily Meal Plan Units

_6-7_ Complete Protein

_8-9_ Fat

_10_ Grain

_3_ Vegetable

_10_ Fruit

_3_ Milk (Skim)

Sample Distribution of Units in Meals and Snacks

MEALS		SNACKS	
_4-5_	Complete Protein	_2_	Complete Protein
_5-6_	Fat	_3_	Fat
_8_	Grain	_2_	Grain
_3_	Vegetable	_0_	Vegetable
_7_	Fruit	_3_	Fruit
_3_	Milk	_0_	Milk

SAMPLE HOME MEAL PLAN — ANOREXIA NERVOSA

	FOOD ITEM	AMOUNT	COMPLETE PROTEIN	FAT	GRAIN	VEGIES	FRUITS	MILK	CUPS OF FLUID
TIME									
B R E A K F A S T	orange juice	1 cup					2		1
	Rice Chex cereal	3/4 cup			1				
	English muffin/marg.	1/1 tsp.		1	2				
	honey	1 Tbsp.					1		
	skim milk	1 cup						1	1
TIME									
L U N C H	SCHOOL LUNCH PROGRAM								
	hamburger patty	2 oz.	2	1					
	hamburger bun				2				
	cooked carrots, plain	1/2 cup				1			
	fresh pear	1					1		
	skim milk	1 cup						1	1
TIME									
S U P P E R	PIZZA HUT RESTAURANT								
	pepperoni thin 'n crispy pizza, medium size	2 slices	2	2	2	2			
	tossed salad from salad bar					1			
	French dressing	1 Tbsp.		1					
	2% milk	1 cup		1				1	1
S N A C K S	AFTERNOON: apple	1 large					2		
	American cheese	2 oz	2	1					
	saltines	6			1				
	EVENING: sugar cookies	2 ave.		2	1		1		
	cranberry juice	1 cup					3		1
	TOTAL NUMBER OF FOOD UNITS		6	9	9	4	10	3	

YOUR MEAL PLAN

Name _MAINTENANCE MEAL PLAN_   Date_____
     (BULIMIA NERVOSA)

Daily Meal Plan Units

_5-7_ Complete Protein

_5_ Fat

_8_ Grain

_1-2_ Vegetable

_4_ Fruit

_1½_ Milk (Skim)

Sample Distribution of Units in Meals and Snacks

MEALS	SNACKS
_3-5_ Complete Protein	_2_ Complete Protein
_4_ Fat	_1_ Fat
_6_ Grain	_2_ Grain
_1-2_ Vegetable	_0_ Vegetable
_3_ Fruit	_1_ Fruit
_1½_ Milk	_0_ Milk

SAMPLE HOME MEAL PLAN — BULIMIA NERVOSA

| FOOD ITEM | AMOUNT | FOOD GROUP | | | | | | |
		COMPLETE PROTEIN	FAT	GRAIN	VEGIES	FRUITS	MILK	CUPS OF FLUID
TIME								
BREAKFAST								
orange juice	½cup					1		½
Rice Krispies cereal	¾cup			1				
toast /margarine	1slice/1tsp		1	1				
jelly	1 Tbsp.					1		
skim milk	½cup						½	½
TIME								
LUNCH								
casserole (any kind)	1cup	2	1	2				
broccoli, cooked	½cup				1			
banana	½ large					1		
skim milk	1cup						1	1
coffee, black	1cup							1
TIME								
SUPPER								
oven-baked chicken leg (with skin, breaded)	2oz	2		½				
baked potato	1small			1				
cooked carrots	½cup				1			
margarine	2 tsp.		2					
dinner roll	1small			1				
mineral water	12 oz							1½
SNACKS EVENING - iced tea	1cup							1
sandwich) roast beef	2oz	2						
bread	2slices			2				
margarine	1tsp		1					
apple	1small					1		
TOTAL NUMBER OF FOOD UNITS		6	5	8½	2	4	1½	5½

SUMMARY OF DSM III-R DIAGNOSTIC CRITERIA FOR ANOREXIA NERVOSA/BULIMIA NERVOSA[12]

Anorexia Nervosa

1. Intense fear of gaining weight or becoming obese while below average body weight standards.

2. Disturbance of body image (e.g., "feeling fat" even when significantly below average body weight standards).

3. Refusal to maintain weight above a minimum expected weight for age and height (below 15% of a minimal normal weight or failure to gain sufficient weight during growth periods).

4. In females, cessation of menses over at least three consecutive months (not caused by other known medical problems).

Bulimia Nervosa

1. Repeated instances of binge eating (rapid intake of large quantities of food in a defined period of time).

2. Weight loss is attempted by one or more purging methods: laxatives, diuretics, vomiting, strict dieting, or excessive exercise.

3. Binge eating is accompanied by a feeling of loss of control over eating.

4. An average minimum frequency of two binge instances per week for at least three months.

5. Ongoing preoccupation with weight and body proportions.

Case Studies

CASE STUDIES

Introduction

Two case studies are presented in order to illustrate the course of weight restoration/stabilization and the nutrition education process. Sample calculations for each of these case studies are included in the *Professional's Guide,* Section III. Corresponding meal plan sheets and menus follow.

The first case study describes the treatment approach used for a patient with anorexia nervosa in a hospital-based eating disorders program. Extensive weight restoration is indicated for this patient.

The second case study illustrates the process of nutrition education for a bulimic patient in a clinic setting where a formalized outpatient eating disorders program does not exist. Weight stabilization is one goal of treatment for this patient.

Anorexia Nervosa — Inpatient Case Study

A. Overview of Program Phases

Based on the model of our inpatient program, treatment is organized into five phases. In the first three phases, some health care team members (the psychiatrist, nurse specialist, occupational therapist) and patient focus on major non-nutritional issues of eating disorders such as self-esteem, assertiveness skills, effective problem-solving techniques, family dynamics, and the three dimensional model of human behavior. The patient's medical status and eating behaviors are closely monitored by the staff.

The dietitian does not work with the patient on a one-to-one basis until the end of the third phase. Throughout the first three phases, meals and snacks are not selected by the patient. Selections are predetermined by the dietitian based on principles of healthy eating and with consideration to general trends in food acceptance (example: roast beef and chicken instead of lamb and liver). Nutrition education in the first three phases is limited to weekly group nutrition classes using *Nutrition for Recovery: Eating Disorders* class outlines.

Individualized meal planning education via extensive review of "Your Home Meal Plan" is reserved for the fourth phase of the hospital program after the patient has attained the vital goals of weight restoration and exposure to healthy eating. In the fifth phase, the home meal plan and other coping strategies are intentionally tested in high-risk situations identified by the patient. At this point the patient is functioning at a highly independent level. The health care team members serve as standby resource people and, as requested by the patient, help to review and enhance coping strategies used in the final program phase.

B. The Patient

A 16-year-old adolescent presented with the diagnosis of anorexia nervosa. Her hospital admission weight was 98 pounds and her height was 66 inches. The patient recalled the duration of restrictive eating to be approximately one year. The patient stated her highest weight to be 130 pounds and lowest weight to be the current weight of 98 pounds. The patient had been weighing herself three to four times daily; her goal was to maintain her weight below 100 pounds. Amenorrhea was noted at a weight of approximately 105 pounds.

The patient denied use of laxatives, diuretics, diet pills, alcohol, or other substance abuse. Her usual daily exercise pattern consisted of running for one hour and biking ten miles although this was becoming more difficult to maintain due to decreasing stamina. The patient's motivation for exercising was to become physically fit and to accelerate weight loss.

Diet History

The patient began to diet following comments from high school peers that she was too fat. For the past three months, food intake was reduced to 700 to 900 calories per day. Variety of selected foods was confined to fresh fruits, raw vegetables, low-fat cottage cheese, soda crackers and diet Pepsi. The patient did not use vitamin-mineral supplements.

Weight Restoration

Treatment goals of the first three phases included restoration of weight and exposure to an increased variety of foods. The initial nonselective diet order was 1200 calories with low lactose, 3 grams of sodium, low fat and six feeding parameters. A multivitamin-mineral supplement was prescribed. The midpoint weight (119 pounds) of the recommended weight range (117 to 122 pounds) was achieved in eight weeks at a weight gain rate of approximately 3 pounds per week. This was accomplished by increasing the nonselective diet by 300 calorie increments (1200 to 1500 to 1800 ...) up to a maximum intake of 4200 calories for this patient.

At the beginning of the third phase of the hospital program, the patient was asked to list eight to ten high-risk (most feared) foods. One of these high-risk foods was sent to the patient daily, while a calorically equivalent menu item or snack item was deleted.

Nutrition Education

Toward the end of the third phase, the patient approached the recommended weight range. The dietitian interviewed the patient regarding anticipated living/schedule aspects such as work or school hours, family involvement with home food preparation/grocery shopping, and the patient's cooking skills. This information was used to develop the home meal plan.

When the patient reached the midpoint weight of 119 pounds and other program criteria were met, she was informed of the recommended weight range and was advanced to the fourth phase. Also, the patient began to select meals and snacks from the regular menu according to her individualized home meal plan. The plan was based upon these factors: an initial weight maintenance calorie requirement of 2500 calories per day, three meals per day (plus snacks per patient preference), representation of all core food groups, a reasonable division of calories into energy nutrients, and the patient's relative comfort level with the core food groups.

In the fourth program phase the patient was asked to write five sample menus according to her meal plan, incorporating variables mentioned during the interview such as fast foods, international foods, school lunch program, and Sunday brunch. These sample menus were checked by the dietitian for accuracy, using the flexibility of three food units above or below the meal plan.

Because the patient had not routinely eaten breakfast prior to admission, scheduled post-discharge mealtimes were planned (breakfast between 7-7:30 a.m. on school days, lunch at school from 12-12:30 p.m. and supper between 5-7:00 p.m. to accommodate her family's usual supper hours).

Throughout hospitalization, the patient attended weekly nutrition group classes. Because of impaired ability to concentrate and participate in group discussion in the first three weeks of hospitalization, it was determined that the patient would benefit from class repetition.

Exercise was limited to program guidelines of 20 to 30 minutes of aerobic exercise per day. Because the patient held an association of weight loss and exercise, the patient was encouraged to maintain reduced amounts of exercise following hospital discharge.

In the last phase of the program, the patient rehearsed coping behaviors in response to anticipated high-risk situations. For example, the patient obtained and ate noon and supper meals in the hospital cafeteria in order to gain more confidence in selecting foods from a cafeteria line and eating in public. The patient joined the family in a restaurant brunch, utilizing her meal plan in eating adequate amounts of foods in this setting. The patient cooked some of her own meals in hospital unit kitchen. In a weight-related risk situation, the patient purchased larger-sized jeans at a shopping mall.

Because both parents shared cooking responsibilities at home, the dietitian led a discussion with the parents and patient to review meal planning recommendations and supportive family roles.

As the patient lived a significant distance from the hospital, the inpatient eating disorders team made arrangements for follow-up with a mental health counselor and dietitian in the patient's home town. After securing written permission from the patient, the inpatient dietitian relayed appropriate information to the home town dietitian regarding weight range, home meal plan, and learned coping strategies to high-risk situations.

The multivitamin-mineral supplement was discontinued at discharge upon consideration of the nutritional adequacy of the home meal plan.

Outpatient Follow-up

Compliance to the meal plan was good; occasional slips of one-day fasting occurred in some stressful situations. These slips were reviewed in light of the analogy of falling off a bicycle. Alternative behavioral strategies were discussed to aid in coping with similar high-risk situations that may occur. Some examples are as follows: (a) Role playing was used by the patient and dietitian as a method to practice the patient's assertiveness skills when confronted with parental pressure to control her food intake. (b) The patient enrolled in a community heart health cooking class in order to become more comfortable with cooking. (c) The patient was encouraged to experiment with eating an unplanned meal when faced with unexpected social occasions such as going out for pizza with friends. The set point theory was used to support this suggestion. Weight was generally maintained within the recommended healthy weight range. The meal plan was not adjusted for isolated minor deviations from the weight range.

After seven months of meal planning and outpatient dietitian follow-up, the patient elected to gradually discontinue meal planning and instead rely upon appetite, regular meal times and learned healthy eating habits. The patient identified progress with long-term personal goals: improved health, higher grades at school, and enhanced interaction with family and friends. These benefits surpassed the patient's occasional desire to renew dieting and weight loss.

Bulimia Nervosa — Outpatient Case Study

General Comments

Initial treatment is attempted in an outpatient psychiatric facility because the patient's medical status is considered sufficiently stable and outpatient therapy is a less costly mode of treatment compared to extended inpatient eating disorders programs.

In this example, a psychologist has requested the collaboration of a dietitian in private practice to provide treatment for the patient. There are no structured program phases in this setting. The psychologist and dietitian schedule separate weekly sessions with the patient in the early course of treatment. After baseline information has been reviewed and the home meal plan begun, follow-up sessions with the dietitian are scheduled every other week. (The frequency of sessions may be adjusted depending on patient status.)

The psychologist and dietitian request the patient to sign a treatment contract which summarizes primary goals such as weight stabilization rather than intentional weight loss, termination of purging and meals consumed on a regular schedule. The contract also provides an acknowledgment for the necessity of ongoing communication between the psychologist and dietitian for purposes of maintaining an effective treatment plan. The dietitian weighs the patient weekly. The psychologist arranges for periodic blood tests to check for electrolyte balance.

The Patient

A 30-year-old woman presented with the diagnosis of bulimia nervosa. Duration of the disorder was three years. Her height was 64 inches and current weight was 135 pounds; significant weight fluctuations were noted by the patient with weight ranging from 120 pounds to 143 pounds. The patient's weight goal was to maintain weight at 100 pounds. The patient recalled a stable predisorder weight of 120 to 125 pounds.

The patient denied use of diuretics, diet pills, alcohol, and illegal substances. Over-the-counter laxatives were used once or twice daily in twice the recommended dosages. Vomiting occurred three to four times per week. Exercise generally consisted of walking for one hour daily. The patient was not receiving any antidepressant medications.

Diet History

The patient resided at a group home with ongoing psychiatric follow-up for depression. Three meals per day were available at the group home. Menus were not posted for the residents. The patient typically did not eat breakfast, would eat lunch only if the entree was a cold sandwich, and did eat a large supper meal consisting of double or triple menu portions. In addition, the patient would frequently consume three to four pastries from a tray of pastries provided in the activities room each morning. When walking in the afternoon, the patient would stop at a convenience store and purchase a large bag of snack chips or cookies to consume on the walk or in the evening.

Nutrition Education

Goals included stabilization of weight (with the weight goal defined as 135 pounds or lower), abandonment of the unrealistic weight goal of 100 pounds, termination of laxative abuse and vomiting, and improvement of eating habits. The focus of eating habits was to eat three meals per day and to enhance the quality of food choices: decreasing intake of sweets and snack chips, and increasing consumption of dairy products, fruits and other complex carbohydrates. The initial outpatient meal plan consisted of 1600 calories with an increase from $1/2$ cup of milk to $1^1/2$ cups of milk per day. (The calorie level of the meal plan was not disclosed to the patient.) A multivitamin-mineral supplement was recommended. At the initial session, sample home menus were jointly written by the patient and dietitian in order to aid the implementation of the meal plan. The patient was seen once a week until the content of the meal planning system was covered, and the patient was able to accurately write home menus via the meal planning system.

The patient was then scheduled weekly for follow-up by the dietitian. Weights were monitored by the dietitian although the patient elected not to know her weights in the first two months of outpatient treatment. The emphasis of the weekly sessions was discussing progress made with healthy eating habits via review of home menus written by the patient. *Nutrition for Recovery* class outlines were covered. High-risk situations that occurred were discussed. The frequency of vomiting and laxative abuse was monitored with the discussion of events or feelings which triggered the actions.

Initial coping strategies were directed toward increasing assertiveness, effective problem-solving and meal planning. Some examples are as follows:

- The patient requested provision of fresh fruit in addition to pastries as a morning snack.

- The morning snack tray was relocated to a less conspicuous place in the activities room.

- An alternative route for afternoon walks was taken to avoid the convenience store.

- The patient requested the manager of the group home to provide menus one week in advance to enable meal planning efforts.

- The patient preferred to eat an evening snack; low-risk foods were planned for this time of day.

Through improved eating habits and assurances that the patient was not gaining weight, use of laxatives and the frequency of vomiting declined to one or two occurrences per week over the first two months of outpatient treatment. This progress was reviewed in context of the learning curve. The meal plan was adjusted upward by 200 calories approximately one month into follow-up in response to the patient experiencing excessive hunger in the late afternoon. Her weight remained stable between 130 to 135 pounds.

Three months into treatment, the patient relapsed in response to a change in relationship with her boyfriend. The patient became noncompliant with the treatment contract. Binging and purging escalated beyond the frequency existing at the outset of treatment. The psychologist and dietitian determined the following response:

- The patient was informed of hazardous medical consequences.

- By breaking the contract, the patient was unable to make reasonable decisions for her well-being.

- The psychologist referred the patient to a physician for close medical monitoring in view of the patient's history and of placing her life at risk. The physician's appointments were scheduled for her. If she failed to come for these appointments, law enforcement officials would be notified to escort the patient to a hospital or facility with a formal inpatient eating disorders program.

- Ongoing consultation with the psychologist and dietitian was canceled. If the patient was willing to abide by the treatment contract, consultation would be resumed.

After approximately six weeks of physician monitoring and one brief hospitalization for rehydration, the patient chose to reattempt counseling with the psychologist and dietitian. From that point on, the patient was generally compliant with treatment. As healthy eating habits and other coping strategies became more established, the patient was able to perceive long-term benefits. These long term benefits included improved health, enhanced self-esteem with less guilt associated with eating, money not spent on laxatives/binge foods was used for recreation, improved social interaction with friends, and a renewed focus on personal long-term goals including future enrollment in college.

Annotated Bibliography

ANNOTATED BIBLIOGRAPHY

Agras, W., Losch, M., Rossiter, E., and Telch, C.: Dietary Restraint of Bulimic Subjects Following Cognitive-Behavioral or Pharmacological Treatment. *Behav. Res. Ther.*, 26: No. 6:495, 1988.

The caloric intake of bulimic patients following treatment with either cognitive-behavioral therapy or imipramine was compared. While both groups of patients decreased their purged calories significantly, only the cognitive-behavioral treatment subjects increased non-purged caloric intake toward a more normal food intake. The imipramine-treated group did not demonstrate a significant increase of non-purged calories, thereby maintaining restricted food intake. The results of this study may help explain superior long-term treatment results following cognitive-behavioral therapy than by pharmacological treatment.

Aughey, D., and Jacobson, K.: What's Eating at Our Youth: Overview of Disordered Eating. *Topics in Pediatrics* (Winter):11, 1988.

This article reviews the following areas of anorexia nervosa and bulimia nervosa: prevalence, diagnostic criteria, medical consequences, early signs of disordered eating and strategies for the health professional in terms of prevention and early intervention.

Bennett, W., and Gurin, J.: *The Dieter's Dilemma*. New York. Basic Books, Inc., 1982.

This book explores the set point theory of weight control. One main premise is that the body will defend its set point of body fat in response to either caloric restriction or caloric excess. Dieting, in most cases, is shown to be counterproductive to weight control because dieting resists, rather than resets, the set point. Throughout the test, numerous metabolic studies are cited. In addition, a historical look at fashion trends/perceptions of beauty are discussed. The reader gains important perspectives regarding the limitations of published "ideal" weight-for-height tables and of the problems associated with accurately predicting energy requirements for any individual. In summary, this text provides valuable insight into many issues regarding dieting and metabolism that arise when counseling individuals with eating disorders. (This book has been made available to our hospitalized patients as optional reading.)

Bolland, J., Bolland, T., and Yuhas, J.: Estimation of Food Portion Sizes: Effectiveness of Training. *J. Am. Diet. Assoc.*, 88:817, 1988.

This study compared the effectiveness of two types of training (food models and household measures) on participants' ability to estimate food portions. These results were then compared with the ability of a control group to estimate portions without training. This study indicates that both training methods improved accuracy in estimating some food portions to a similar degree. (Both methods are used as an optional activity in the class *Nutrition Know How: Introduction to Meal Planning*. Class participants are asked to identify food models with food groups and to estimate portions of actual foods to units indicated in the meal planning system.)

Bouchard, C., Despres, J., Dussault, J., Fournier, G., Lupien, P., Morrjani, S., Nadeau, A., Pinault, S., Theriault, G., Treblay, A.: The Response to Long-Term Overfeeding in Identical Twins. *N. Engl. J. Med.*, 322:1477, 1990.

This study of overfeeding in 12 pairs of identical twins helps to explain why some people maintain weight with unrestricted food intake while other people are prone to weight gain on food intake not markedly above energy needs.

During 12 weeks of overfeeding, each individual consumed 1000 calories per day above estimated weight maintenance energy needs. At the conclusion of the overfeeding period, some individuals had significant weight increases (up to 29 pounds). Other individuals experienced relatively small weight gain; the lowest weight gain was 9 pounds. A genetic influence is strongly supported in that there was three times more variation in body weight, body composition and body energy content between pairs than within pairs.

Brewer, M., Hegsted, M., Howat, P., Mills, G., and Varner, L.: The Effect of Bulimia Upon Diet, Body Fat, Bone Density, and Blood Components. *J. Am. Diet. Assoc.*, 89:929, 1989.

Blood components, bone mineral density and percentage of body fat were compared between eight bulimic women and 10 control women. Mean age, height and weight of participants were similar. Percentage of body fat was similar. Menstrual dysfunction was experienced by three bulimic women. 100% of the control women and 13% of the bulimic women were on multivitamins with minerals. Folacin intake was significantly lower in the bulimic women. Mean intake of calcium exceeded 800 milligrams for all women. Bone mineral density was lower in bulimic subjects. The lowest bone density was found in a woman with a 26 year history of bulimia. It appears that extent of decreased bone density is associated with the duration and intensity of purging behaviors.

Dietz. W., and Hartung, R.: Changes in Height Velocity of Obese Preadolescents During Weight Reduction. *Am. J. D. C.*, 139:705, 1985.

Changes in the rate of linear growth before and during a nine month period of weight reduction were studied in 19 obese preadolescents. The caloric intake was reduced to approximately two-thirds of the usual daily intake. Protein intake was maintained at 1.5 to 2.0 grams per kilogram of ideal body weight. This study confirms that height velocity was significantly reduced during the nine month period in which the children were following balanced, mild calorie-deficit diets. Long-term implications are not known. There is no evidence to suggest that a short-term slowing of linear growth in obese children results in permanent stunting. This study indicates the need for monitoring growth rates of children who are dieting. An area of future research is to determine an optimal weight reduction diet that will not impede linear growth rate.

Ebert, M., George, T., Gwirtsman, H., Jimerson, D., Kaye, W., and Obarzanek, E.: Caloric Intake Necessary for Weight Maintenance in Anorexia Nervosa: Nonbulimics Require Greater Caloric Intake than Bulimics. *Am. J. Clin. Nutr.*, 44:435, 1986.

This study compared caloric intake needed to stabilize weight between bulimic anorectics and nonbulimic anorectics. It was found that nonbulimic anorectics required 30 to 50% more calories to sustain weight at various stages of refeeding than bulimic anorectics.

A second finding is that short-term weight restored anorectics needed more calories to maintain a stable weight than long-term weight restored anorectics. More longitudinal studies are needed to support this observation.

Clinical significance of these results: nonbulimic anorectics will have greater difficulty in maintaining weight because of the quantity of food needed coupled with a less efficient energy metabolism. In contrast, bulimic anorectics are at risk for obesity due to a more efficient metabolism.

Ebert, M., George, T., Gwirtsman, H., Kaye, W., and Petersen, R.: Caloric Consumption and Activity Levels After Weight Recovery in Anorexia Nervosa: A Prolonged Delay in Normalization. *Int. J. Eating Disorders*, 5:No. 3:503, 1986.

Groups of anorectic patients were studied for caloric intake necessary to maintain healthy weight following refeeding. In the short-term period following refeeding (2 to 6 weeks), patients had significantly greater intake of calories than did long-term (6 months) weight-recovered anorectics. In addition, the short-term weight-recovered anorectics had elevated levels of activity when compared to the long-term weight-recovered anorectics. While increased activity may account in part for increased calorie requirements, it is speculated that there may be a delay in the normalization of several neuroendocrine systems involved in metabolism.

The implications of this study is that weight-recovered anorectics will benefit from nutritional/meal planning follow-up well beyond short-term weight recovery and that patients may be advised to expect increased food intake for several months.

Fogelman, I., Murby, B., Russell, G., and Treasure, J.: Reversible Bone Loss in Anorexia Nervosa. *Br. Med. J.*, 295:474, 1987.

Four groups of subjects were assessed for bone mineral density in the lumbar spine, hip and wrist. The groups consisted of 45 active anorectics, with ages 14 to 54 who had fallen to a minimum of 75% of their usual weight and had amenorrhea for over a year, 31 healthy control subjects with similar ages, 25 recovered anorectics with ages 23 to 52 and 20 age-matched healthy control subjects.

Bone density for all active anorectics had decreased in proportion to the duration of illness. For all 20 patients whose amenorrhea was of six years or more, bone density of the hip site was two standard deviations below the mean. Fracture had occurred in nine patients; of these patients eight had suffered from anorexia nervosa for over 10 years.

Bone density improved for subjects recovering from their disorder in response to weight gain. This response occurred prior to the return of menses. Bone density was normal in subjects who had recovered from the disorder.

Friedman, M.: Metabolic Control of Food Intake. *Contemporary Nutrition,* 13:No. 7, 1988.

This article summarizes current thinking regarding metabolic signals that regulate intake of food. A long held theory is that a twofold system exists: A glucostatic signal and a lipostatic signal that are integrated via neural mediation.

A second theory reviewed is that intracellular oxidation of glucose and fat provides a signal detected by the liver. Hepatic control may influence sensory food preferences in addition to amounts of food consumed. The possibility is raised that dietary fat calories may bypass metabolic control of food intake because they are readily stored as adipose tissue. This theory provides an explanation for overeating in the dynamic stage of obesity and overeating in response to high fat diets.

Frisch, R., and McArthur, J.: Menstrual Cycles: Fatness as a Determinant of Minimum Weight for Height Necessary for their Maintenance or Onset. *Science,* 185:949, 1974.

This article provides a method of estimating a minimal weight for height necessary for the onset of menses in primary amenorrhea due to food restriction and for restoration of menses in secondary amenorrhea due to food restriction.

Women of ages 16 and over with secondary amenorrhea resumed menses at a heavier weight (equivalent to approximately 22 percent fat of body weight) than the weight of menarche of girls with primary amenorrhea (equivalent to approximately 17 percent fat of body weight). These standards apply only to Caucasian United States and European females since different races have different critical weights at menarche. These standards are shown on page 20 of the "Professional's Guide."

Other factors, including emotional stress, affect menses. Therefore, amenorrhea may occur in the absence of weight loss and menses may not resume in some individuals even when minimal weight is attained.

Garfinkel, P., and Garner, D.: *Handbook of Psychotherapy for Anorexia and Bulimia*. New York. The Guilford Press, 1985.

This book is considered to be a primary reference on eating disorders. Various treatment approaches are reviewed, including behavioral, cognitive, family, group and psychotherapy. Three chapters have been of particular interest in developing our eating disorders program: Chapter 14 "Inpatient Treatment for Anorexia Nervosa," Chapter 15 "Special Problems of Inpatient Management," and Chapter 21 "Psychoeducational Principles in the Treatment of Bulimia and Anorexia Nervosa."

Chapter 21 has been a required reading for all patients in the first phase of our inpatient program. This chapter deals with cultural pressures to be thin, metabolic adaptation to dieting, set point theory, ineffectiveness of purging, physical complications of eating disorders and healthy eating parameters.

Hall, R., and Hooker, C.: Nutritional Assessment of Patients with Anorexia and Bulimia; Clinical and Laboratory Findings. *Psychiatric Med* 7:No. 3:27, 1989.

The process of nutritional assessment conducted in a 13-bed inpatient eating disorders unit is reviewed. Included is a commentary on the usefulness of anthropometric measurements and laboratory values. A sample dietary questionnaire is included.

Ireton-Jones, C., and Sedlet, K.: Energy Expenditure and the Abnormal Eating Pattern of a Bulimic: A Case Report. *J. Am. Assoc.* 89:74, 1989.

Studies have shown that basal metabolic rate is reduced in bulimic patients. Elevated energy efficiency may increase the likelihood of purging behaviors as an attempt to counteract weight gain. Increased energy efficiency may be a result of chronic dieting.

In this study, estimated basal energy expenditure (BEE) using the Harris-Benedict equation and measured energy expenditure (MEE) was determined of a bulimic individual before and after normalization of her eating pattern. Her BEE (1266 kcal) was significantly higher than her MEE (829 kcal) while alternating binge eating/purging and semifasting behaviors. Following normalization of eating, there was a 50 percent increase of her MEE which was similar to the calculated BEE.

It is important to convey to patients that bulimic behaviors may slow metabolic rate and that resumption of healthy eating patterns will normalize metabolic rate.

Keesey, R.: The Body-Weight Set Point: What Can You Tell Your Patients? *Postgrad. Med.*, 83:114, 1988.

This article provides an update on the set point theory of weight regulation. From animal studies, it has been shown that obesity may be genetically transmitted and metabolically defended. This may support the finding that many obese people eat no more than lean people. Obesity may be diet-induced: with prolonged intake of a high fat diet, metabolic resistance to weight gain can be overcome. In this case, the new elevated set point will be defended. Obesity may also be induced by damage to the hypothalamus. This type of obesity is not regulated, or defended by alterations in metabolism.

Research on human obesity raises the possibility that both regulated and unregulated types of obesity exist. If obesity appears to be regulated as evidenced by strong metabolic defense, sustained weight reduction will be very difficult to achieve. Long-term dieting, as well as suboptimal nutrition, may be too high a price to pay for weight loss.

Future research may reveal means to effectively alter elevated body-weight set point.

Krey, S., Palmer, K., and Porcelli, K.: Eating Disorders: The Clinical Dietitian's Changing Role. *J. Am. Diet. Assoc.*, 89:41, 1989.

Consensus exists that most patients require a multidisciplinary approach that concurrently addresses both physiological and psychological aspects of eating disorders. The clinical dietitian plays a vital role in achieving patient goals of restoring nutritional health and maintaining healthy eating patterns. Nutritional rehabilitation will involve both short-term and long-term goals, either in a combination of both inpatient and outpatient treatment or solely outpatient treatment.

Nash, J.: Eating Behavior and Body Weight: Physiological Influences. *Am. J. Health Promotion*, 1(3):5, 1987.

This overview focuses on physiological influences involved with body weight. Heredity plays an important role; however, it is not equated with destiny for most people. According to the fat cell theory, early onset hyperplastic obesity is more resistant to change. Therefore, prevention and intervention of obesity is more effective in childhood and in adolescence.

Other topics presented include: arguments for and against the set point theory, brown fat cell theory, effect of macronutrient distribution, and the metabolic benefit of small frequent feedings in contrast to large infrequent feedings.

Many physiological aspects influence eating behaviors, which along with exercise, determine body weight. Psychosocial factors also impact upon eating behaviors which are discussed in the accompanying article, "Eating Behavior and Body Weight: Psychosocial Influences."

Nash, J.: Eating Behavior and Body Weight: Psychosocial Influences. *Am J Health Promotion*, 1:5, 1987.

Psychological, social and cultural influences on eating behavior and body weight are reviewed. When considered with physiological influences, obesity is a very complex condition. Voluntary weight reduction is difficult to achieve for many people.

Topics reviewed include personality traits, emotional states, external food-related cues, behavior modification, cognitive restructuring and cultural pressures for thinness.

Based on physiological and psychosocial influences reviewed, ten recommendations for treatment of obesity are provided. Some of these recommendations include: help the client to reeducate taste preferences, provide social skills training (assertiveness, conflict resolution), expand nutrition education, emphasize an exercise component and provide relapse prevention techniques.

Newsholme, E.: A Possible Metabolic Basis for the Control of Body Weight. *N. Engl. J. Med.*, 302:400, 1980.

Both body weight and metabolism may be regulated in part by substrate cycling. A substrate cycle exists when a forward reaction in a metabolic pathway is opposed by a separate reaction in the reverse direction of the pathway. Cycling produces chemical energy which is dissipated in the form of heat. By this means, excess calories may be burned off.

It is speculated that obesity may result, in part, from a low capacity of substrate cycles in tissues or an impairment of hormonal mechanisms that control the rate of substrate cycling.

<u>References</u>

REFERENCES

1. Gordon, J., and Marlatt, G. A., Eds., *Relapse Prevention: Maintenance Strategies in the Treatment of Addiction*, The Guilford Press, New York, 1985.

2. *The Waist Land: Why Diets Don't Work* (videotape). Coronet/MTI Film and Video, 108 Wilmont Road, Deerfield, Illinois 60015. Phone 1-800-621-2131.

3. Nasco Nutrition Teaching Aids (food replicas catalog). Nasco, 901 Janesville Avenue, Fort Atkinson, Wisconsin 53538-0901. Phone 1-800-558-9595.

4. Metropolitan Life Insurance Company Height/Weight Data: Statistical Bulletin. Vol. 64, No. 1, 6, 1959.

5. Frisch, R., and McArthur, J., Menstrual Cycles: Fatness as a Determinant of Minimum Weight for Height Necessary for their Maintenance or Onset, *Science*, 185, 949, 1974.

6. Food and Nutrition Board, National Academy of Sciences - National Research Council, *Recommended Dietary Allowances*, National Academy Press, Washington, D. C., 1989.

7. American Diabetes Association, Inc., and American Dietetic Association, *Exchange Lists for Meal Planning*, 1989.

8. Canadian Diabetes Association: *Good Health Eating Guide*, 1990.

9. Katch, F. and McArdle, W., *Nutrition, Weight Control and Exercise*, 2nd Ed., Lea and Febiger, Philadelphia, 1983, 308.

10. Marcus, J. (Ed.), *Sports Nutrition — A Guide for the Professional Working with Active People*, The American Dietetic Association, Chicago, 1986, 141.

11. Adapted from "Healthy Eating — A Meal Planning System," University of Minnesota, Minneapolis, 1987.

12. American Psychiatric Association, *Diagnostic and Statistical Manual of Mental Disorders*, Third Edition — Revised, Washington, D. C., 1987, 67–69.

YOUR HOME MEAL PLAN

ACKNOWLEDGMENTS

I wish to thank the following people for their review and suggestions:

David Abbott, M.D., Co-Director, MeritCare Eating Disorders Program/Director, St. Luke's Hospitals MeritCare Inpatient Eating Disorders Program

Debra Nelson, R.N., B.S.N., Coordinator, MeritCare Eating Disorders Program

Linda Schander, L.R.D., MeritCare Eating Disorders Program

Stephen Wonderlich, Ph.D., Co-Director, MeritCare Eating Disorders Program; Associate Professor, Department of Psychiatry, University of North Dakota, School of Medicine

In addition, I wish to acknowledge the important feedback and suggestions offered by patients of the MeritCare Inpatient Eating Disorders Program, St. Luke's Hospitals MeritCare, Fargo, North Dakota.

I appreciate the assistance given by many restaurant and food companies in providing nutrition information about their products.

I. INTRODUCTION

Recovery is dependent upon an intake of food that is adequate in amount and quality. An important goal of meal planning is to provide a definition of how to achieve healthy eating through a wide variety of foods. Your maintenance calorie level is a prediction based upon such variables as your height, target weight range, age and anticipated home activity level. Your maintenance calorie level may be adjusted by your outpatient dietitian or doctor if your weight consistently falls above or below the target weight range. If you are 16 years of age or younger, your calorie level and target weight range may increase to allow for growth.

Quality aspects of meal planning are based upon the 1990 edition of "Dietary Guidelines for Americans".[1] A focus of these guidelines is to recommend a healthy distribution of the three energy-carrying nutrients: carbohydrate, protein and fat. Your home meal plan includes a healthy distribution of these nutrients.

Set Point Theory and Meal Planning — Connections

The set point theory suggests that each person has a unique stable adult weight range and percentage of body fat. The body is capable of maintaining a stable weight range while a person is practicing healthy eating habits and exercise habits. A second interpretation of the set point theory is that the body has an energy set point. Through the action of many internal regulators, the body cares about how many calories it takes in. The goal of the energy set point is a stable range of caloric intake every day. From this theory, which indicates that the body plays the primary role in self weight regulation, several conclusions can be made in regard to meal planning.

1. The body does not demand a precise intake of calories each day; a stable weight range is maintained despite minor fluctuations in day-to-day intake. Therefore, your meal plan does not make direct reference to the caloric value, foods are grouped together based on their similar carbohydrate, protein and fat content. This allows the dietitian to recommend a home meal plan which provides a healthy distribution of these energy-carrying nutrients.

2. Since the body is capable of maintaining a stable weight range with some variation of caloric intake, your meal plan can allow for flexibility in a number of ways:

    a. *Estimating food portions* — Complete protein units are usually given as a range of recommended units such as five to seven units per day. This range is intended to make you more comfortable in visually estimating meat portions by referring to drawings of common meat portions included in your meal planning materials. It is advised that you avoid weighing meats since this is impractical and is also an unnecessary degree of precision.

        You may choose to measure foods found in other groups during the first week following discharge from the hospital or during the first week of outpatient treatment. This will enable you to gain a sense of how common food portions appear in proportion to your drinking glasses, cereal bowls and dinner plates. Thereafter, trust your ability to visually estimate food portions without measuring them. See Figure 1 and Figure 2.

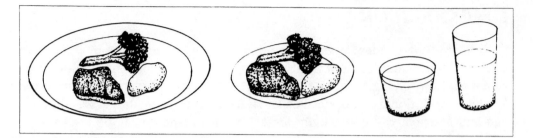

FIGURE 1. Food Portions in Proportion to Dinner Ware.

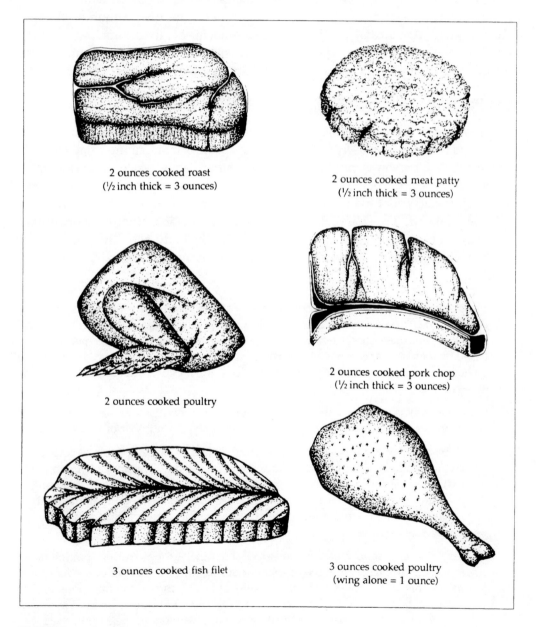

2 ounces cooked roast
(½ inch thick = 3 ounces)

2 ounces cooked meat patty
(½ inch thick = 3 ounces)

2 ounces cooked poultry

2 ounces cooked pork chop
(½ inch thick = 3 ounces)

3 ounces cooked fish filet

3 ounces cooked poultry
(wing alone = 1 ounce)

FIGURE 2. Complete Proteins — Portion Guidelines.

b. *Going above or below your meal plan* — When writing your daily home menus, you may allow some room for flexibility by choosing up to three units above or below your meal plan. Please note however, that this is a two-way street! Continually eating below or above your plan will raise the possibility that your weight may fall out of the recommended weight range. Therefore, on some days it is acceptable to be one to three units below your plan; then on other days try to eat one to three units above your plan in order to be eating up to the meal plan over time. For special events such as an occasional restaurant meal or family celebration, you may choose to eat foods without specifically counting them according to your meal plan. As long as you do not skip meals before or after the special occasion meal, your body can readily handle spontaneous eating without resulting in abrupt weight changes.

c. *Accuracy and simplicity* — Consideration has been given to representing the carbohydrate, protein and fat content of foods as accurately as possible while avoiding difficulty in using the system. For example, the complete protein group has been subdivided into three subgroups in order to present reasonable accuracy. In order to simplify the system, fractions of food units have been almost completely avoided by rounding up or down to the closest whole number. This is another illustration of how the body is able to maintain a stable weight range even with the reality of minor variations of caloric intake from day to day.

The Body's Need for Water

Most adults need 2 to 3 quarts of water each day in order to carry on such vital body processes as the transportation of nutrients to cells, regulation of temperature and elimination of waste products. Almost half of this requirement is obtained from water present in solid foods. The remaining amount of water needed by the body is furnished by drinking 4 to 6 cups of beverages each day. The following list of beverages will contribute toward meeting your daily water requirement:

> bouillon, broth
> carbonated beverages
> decaffeinated coffee
> decaffeinated tea
> herbal tea
> juice
> milk
> mineral water
> regular coffee, if consumed routinely and in moderation
> regular tea, if consumed routinely and in moderation
> water

Certain situations can increase your body's need for water. Some examples include strenuous exercise, fever and prolonged exposure to hot weather. Failure to meet the body's need for water can result in dehydration. As you continue to establish healthy eating habits, it is helpful to assess if you are drinking an adequate amount of fluid each day. If you customarily drink a much larger amount of beverages listed above without the body needing extra fluids, be attentive that frequent consumption of these beverages do not interfere with your ability to eat the recommended amounts of your meal plan units.

Caffeine

The most common sources of caffeine include coffee, tea, chocolate and cola. In addition, certain medications such as some pain relievers and cold preparations contain significant amounts of caffeine.

Caffeine is best known for its stimulant effect. Most adults can consume up to 300 milligrams of caffeine per day (equivalent to approximately 3 cups of brewed coffee) and achieve the "pick-me-up" effect without harm. Although tolerance to caffeine varies among people, increasing intake measurably beyond this level can lead to unpleasant symptoms of anxiety, irritability, sleep disturbances and dryness of the mouth.[2] It is widely accepted that caffeine can aggravate existing ulcers, hiatal hernia and the sensation of heartburn.[2] At present, there is no consistent evidence that links common levels of caffeine intake with cancer and atherosclerosis.

You may be advised to restrict caffeine intake in order to help stabilize fluid balance and avoid any negative effects upon mood and sleep. If you choose to drink caffeinated beverages, a moderate level of caffeine intake (up to approximately 300 milligrams per day) is recommended.

Beverage containing caffeine	Milligrams of caffeine
brewed coffee, 8 oz.	100–150
instant coffee, 8 oz.	85–100
decaffeinated coffee, 8 oz.	2–4
tea, 8 oz.	60–75
cocoa, 8 oz.	5–40
cola drinks, 12 oz.	40–60

Miscellaneous

The food groups shown in *Nutrition for Recovery*, are based upon the American Diabetes Association and American Dietetics Associations' *Exchange Lists for Meal Planning*.[3]

When referring to combination foods, international foods, restaurant foods and frozen entrees groups, Subgroup 2 complete proteins have been used in the calculations unless otherwise indicated. Therefore, fat units can be counted as shown for these food groups in the following sections, Food Groups.

Specific brand names of some products have been listed throughout the meal planning system. Other brands of similar products may be substituted for specific products mentioned.

Various reduced calorie and "lite" products are listed throughout the food groups. Because an important goal of recovery is to avoid a mindset of dieting, the use of those diet-associated products is not encouraged. However, in recognition that these products are available in growing numbers, information is included.

Establishing a Home Eating Schedule

It is extremely important to eat three meals each day at fairly consistent intervals in order to reestablish normal appetite and also to avoid an excessive buildup of hunger - a strong risk factor for binging. Snacks are optional. For the person recovering from anorexia, snacks are helpful in distributing meal plan units throughout the day and in moderating the size of meals. For the person recovering from bulimia, low-risk foods eaten as snacks may be helpful in preventing excessive hunger between meals. In early phases of outpatient treatment for bulimia, it may be wise to avoid former binge foods at high-risk times of the day. As recovery continues, these foods may be gradually introduced.

Recovery

Many patients rely on using the meal plan for three to six months as part of ongoing recovery. Following the meal plan over this time period enables the body to reestablish reliable hunger signals and allows healthy eating to become an automatic habit. You and your outpatient counselors will decide when the time has come for experimenting with eating meals and snacks according to appetite without following your meal plan.

A realistic perspective of recovery is essential. Because many complex behaviors, feelings and thoughts are part of the eating disorder, recovery involves hard work and time. It is likely that recovery will not run a smooth, perfect course. On occasion, a person may "slip" or stumble when confronted with a stressful situation and resort to a binge or a day of fasting. A "slip" (mistake) can be viewed as a *single, temporary fall* from recovery, but not a disaster that can never be undone.[4] It is important to allow room for slips. Slips are not failures; one can even benefit from them. A slip can provide useful information about a stressful situation and may help in planning effective coping actions in the future.[4]

Relapse can be viewed as a series of events or slips that may be followed by a return to recovery or to previous eating disordered behavior.[4] The earlier a person effectively responds to a chain of events leading to a high-risk situation or series of slips, the easier it will be to prevent relapse.[4] Effective responses may include a decision to avoid the high-risk situation or to make advance plans about how to deal with it when it occurs.

When a slip occurs, one can be prepared to cope with it, accept it, learn from it and proceed on track with recovery.

These concepts regarding relapse and slips can be compared with the experience of learning to ride a bicycle. For most people, practice is necessary. A person may occasionally "fall off." The goal is to get back on the bicycle and persist in improving one's balance and skill.[4]

Even after healthy eating habits are well established, you may wish to keep your meal planning materials on file in the event a stressful situation occurs. Following the meal plan during stressful times may reduce the chance of relapse and prove to be an effective coping skill. If a slip or relapse occurs, return to eating according to your meal plan as soon as possible. Your body can forgive a brief slip of unhealthy eating and resume normal metabolic functioning with healthy eating.

II. FOOD GROUPS

A. Core Food Groups

Food Group: Complete Protein (Subgroup 1)

Foods in this subgroup contribute high quality protein and low amounts of fat to your meal plan. Consider the following guidelines when including these foods in your meal plan:

1. One unit is equal to any of the foods listed below.

2. When meats are indicated by ounces, this refers to cooked weight with bone and visible fat removed.

3. These selections are lower in fat value than complete protein foods in Subgroup 2. Therefore, it is appropriate to eat one extra fat unit beyond the total number of fat units recommended in your meal plan for every two to three units of complete protein from this list. Example: A meal plan includes eight fat units per day. If 2 ounces of chicken without skin are eaten, then include nine fat units for that day.

4. Cooking methods include broiling, boiling, baking and roasting.

5. If butter, margarine, oil or shortening is used in cooking, you may count the food as coming from complete protein (Subgroup 2). Example: 2 ounces of cod cooked in butter equals two units of complete protein (Subgroup 2).

6. If the meat has been breaded, add one-half grain unit for every two to three units of cooked meat.

Beef (USDA Good or Choice grade)	1 oz.
Chipped beef	
Flank steak	
Round steak	
Sirloin steak	
Stew meat	
Tenderloin	
Very lean ground beef (90% lean)	
Fish	
All fresh or frozen fish	1 oz.
Clams, crab, lobster	1 oz. or $\frac{1}{3}$ cup
Herring, not creamed	1 oz.
Oysters	6 medium
Sardines, canned in oil, drained	2 medium
Scallops	
Bay, 60–80 raw per pound	6
Large, 20–30 raw per pound	2
Jumbo, less than 20 raw per pound	1
Shrimp	
Colossal, less than 10 raw per pound	1
Jumbo, 16–20 raw per pound	2

Large, 26–35 raw per pound	3
Medium, 51–60 raw per pound	5
Tuna, canned in water	¼ cup
Pork	
Low-fat ham	1 oz.
Poultry	1 oz.
Chicken, without skin	
Cornish hen, without skin	
Turkey, without skin	
Turkey ham	
Veal	
All varieties except for veal cutlets	1 oz.
Wild Game	1 oz.
Duck, without skin	
Goose, without skin	
Pheasant, without skin	
Venison	
Cheese	
Cottage cheese, lowfat or 2%	¼ cup
Diet cheese	1 oz.
Borden Lite Line	
Kraft Free Singles - Nonfat Process	
Cheese Product (count as /2 skim milk)	
Light 'n Lively	
Weight Watcher's Lo-Fat Cheese Slices	
Pot Cheese	¼ cup
Other	
Egg whites	3
Egg substitute	½ cup
95% fat-free luncheon meat	1 oz.

Food Group: Complete Protein (Subgroup 2)

Foods in this subgroup provide high quality protein and moderate amounts of fat to your meal plan. Consider the following guidelines when including these foods in your meal plan:

1. One unit is equal to any of the foods listed below.

2. When meats are indicated by ounces, this refers to cooked weight with bone and visible fat removed.

3. Cooking methods include broiling, boiling, baking and roasting.

4. If butter, margarine, oil or shortening is used in cooking, for every two to three units of any food listed below you may count the food as two to three units of complete protein (Subgroup 2) and one fat unit.

   Example: 3 ounces pork chop fried in oil equals three units of complete protein (Subgroup 2) and one fat unit.

5. If the meat has been breaded, add one-half grain unit for every two to three units of cooked meat.

6. Frankfurters are listed separately at the end of this subgroup.

Beef   1 oz.
    Most beef products are in this subgroup.
    Lean ground beef, 85% lean
    Meatloaf
    Roast (chuck, rib, rump)
    Steak (chuck, cubed, Porterhouse, ribeye, T-bone)
Fish
    Anchovy, drained   9 fillets
    Salmon, canned and drained   1/4 cup
    Tuna, canned in oil and drained   1/4 cup
Lamb   1 oz.
    Most lamb products are in this subgroup.
    Chops
    Roast
Pork   1 oz.
    Most fresh pork products are in this subgroup.
    Chops
    Roast
Poultry   1 oz.
    Chicken with skin
    Duck with skin
    Goose with skin
Veal
    Cutlet, not breaded   1 oz.
Cheese
    Alpine Lace (Colbi-Lo, Monti-Jack-Lo, Provo-Lo)   1 oz.
    Borden's Skim American   1 oz.
    Cheese Kisses   1 oz.
    Cheese Whiz spread   1 oz.
    Creamed cottage cheese, 4% milkfat   1/4 cup
    Farmers   1 oz.
    Kraft Light & Natural (Cheddar, Colby, Swiss)   1 oz.
    Mozzarella   1 oz.
    Neufchatel   1 oz.
    Parmesan   1 oz. or 3 Tbsp. grated
    Ricotta   1/4 cup
    Skim or part-skim milk cheeses   1 oz.
    String cheese   1 oz.
Other
    Egg   2 small or 1 large/jumbo
    86% fat-free luncheon meat   1 oz.
    Lean Supreme Smoked Sausage   1 oz.
    Liver   1 oz.
    Tofu   3 oz. or 2 1/2" x 2 1/2" x 1"
    Wilson 25% Less Fat Smoked Sausage   1 oz.
Frankfurters
    One Hormel Light & Lean 90% Fat Free Frankfurter equals one complete protein.
    One chicken or turkey frankfurter equals one complete protein and one fat unit.
    One Oscar Mayer Light 80% Fat Free Frank equals one complete protein and one fat unit.
    One regular frankfurter equals one complete protein and two fat units.
    One Butterball Bun-Size Turkey Frankfurter equals one complete protein and one fat unit.
    One regular bun-size frankfurter equals one complete protein and two fat units.

Food Group: *Complete Protein (Subgroup 3)*

These foods contribute high quality protein and a higher amount of fat than complete protein (Subgroups 1 and 2). Consider the following guidelines when including these foods into your meal plan:

1. One unit is equal to any of the foods listed below.

2. When meats are indicated by ounces, this refers to cooked weight with bone and visible fat removed.

3. Because these foods are relatively high in fat value, you may use one less fat unit in your meal plan for every two to three units of complete protein chosen from this subgroup.

    Example: A meal plan includes six fat units per day. If 2 ounces of Velveeta cheese are eaten, the cheese may be counted as two units of complete protein (Subgroup 2) and one of the six fat units for that day.

4. Cooking methods include broiling, boiling, baking and roasting.

5. If butter, margarine, oil or shortening is used in cooking, you may count two to three units of food as two to three units of complete protein (Subgroup 3) and one fat unit. The following example will illustrate guidelines 3 and 5.

    Example: A meal plan includes eight fat units per day. If 2 ounces of Spam (fried in oil) are eaten, the Spam may be counted as two units of complete protein (Subgroup 2) and two of the eight fat units for that day.

6. If the meat has been breaded, add one-half grain unit for every two to three units of cooked meat.

Beef	1 oz.
Most cuts of Prime grade are in this subgroup.	
Brisket	
Corned beef brisket	
Ribs	
Rib roast	
Sirloin	
Regular ground beef (80% or less lean)	
Lamb	1 oz.
Breast	
Ground	
Pork	1 oz.
Country style ham	
Deviled ham	
Ground pork	
Sausage	
Spareribs	
Breakfast sausage links	1 1/2 links
Cheese	
All regular cheeses	1 oz.
American	
Bleu	

Cheddar	
Colby	
Monterey Jack	
Muenster	
Provolone	
Swiss	
Alpine Lace (American, Cheddar flavored, Swiss-Lo)	1 oz.
Kraft Extra Thick American Singles	1 slice (1.2 oz.)
Velveeta	1 oz.

See Figure 2, Complete Proteins - Portion Guidelines

Food Group: FAT (Polyunsaturated)

These foods are sources of essential fatty acids and fat-soluble vitamins. In addition, these foods aid in stabilizing your appetite between meals since they are digested at a slower rate than carbohydrate and protein. A moderate intake of fat, especially from the polyunsaturated choices shown on this page, is appropriate for heart health and cancer prevention.

Fat units are often incorrectly thought of as "fattening." When eaten in the amounts shown in your meal plan, fat units provide the benefits stated above and are not "fattening."

One unit is equal to any of the following items.

Avocado	2 Tbsp.
Cooking oil	1 tsp.
Margarine	1 tsp.
Margarine, diet, reduced calorie or light	1 Tbsp.
Nuts and seeds	
Almonds, dry roasted	6 whole
Cashews, dry roasted	5 whole
Chopped nuts	1 Tbsp.
Mixed nuts	4-6 nuts
Peanuts	20 small or 10 large
Pecans	2 whole
Walnuts	2 whole or 1 Tbsp., chopped
Other nuts	1 Tbsp.
Pumpkin seeds	2 tsp.
Seeds, pine nuts, sunflower (without shells)	1 Tbsp.
Olives	10 small or 5 large
Salad dressings	
Buttermilk or milk recipe (Hidden Valley Ranch)	1 Tbsp.
Creamy-type (Thousand Island, Roquefort), *regular*	2 tsp.
Creamy-type (Thousand Island, Roquefort), *reduced calorie*	1 Tbsp.
French, Creamy Italian, Italian, *regular*	1 Tbsp.
French, Creamy Italian, Italian, *reduced calorie*	2 Tbsp.
Mayonnaise or Miracle Whip, *regular*	1 tsp.
Mayonnaise or Miracle Whip, *reduced calorie*	1 Tbsp.
Tartar sauce	1 Tbsp.

Food Group: Fat (Saturated)

Bacon	1 strip
Bacon fat	1 tsp.
Butter	1 tsp.
Coconut, shredded	2 Tbsp.
Coffee whitener	
Liquid	2 Tbsp.
Powder	4 tsp.
Powder, light	2 Tbsp.
Cream cheese	1 Tbsp.
Cream cheese, light	4 tsp.
Cream, heavy	1 Tbsp.
Cream, light (half & half)	2 Tbsp.
Gravy	2 Tbsp.
Light Sour Cream	2 Tbsp.
Sour Cream	1 1/2 Tbsp.
Whipped Cream	1/4 cup
Whipped topping, frozen	3 Tbsp.
Whipped topping, Dzerta mix prepared	1/4 cup
Sauces	
Cheese sauce	1 Tbsp.
Hollandaise sauce	1 Tbsp.
White sauce	2 Tbsp.

Food Group: Grain

A variety of foods are included in this group such as breads, cereals and some vegetables. These foods provide complex carbohydrate and fiber. In addition, grains are an important source of B vitamins and some essential minerals such as iron, magnesium and zinc.

One unit is equal to any of the following items. When adding a unit from the fat group to a grain unit, remember to count the fat unit in your meal plan. For example, one small baked potato eaten with 1 teaspoon margarine equals one grain and one fat unit.

Bread	
White (including French, Italian)	1 slice
Whole wheat	1 slice
Thin-sliced bread	2 slices
"Less" or "lite" bread	2 slices
Raisin, unfrosted	1 slice
Rye, pumpernickel	1 slice
Bagel, any style	1/2
Bread sticks, crisp, (4" long x 1/2")	2
Croutons	1/2 cup
Dough, pretzel, 2 1/2 oz.	1/2
English muffin, any style	1/2
Frankfurter or hamburger bun, medium	1/2
Kaiser roll, small	1
Pita, 6" across	1/2

Plain roll, small	1
Soft breadsticks, Pillsbury	1
Tortilla, 6" across	1

Cereals (Dry)

Bran cereals

All Bran	$1/3$ cup
Bran Buds	$1/3$ cup
40% Bran Flakes	$2/3$ cup
Corn Bran	$1/2$ cup
Cracklin' Oat	$1/3$ cup
Fiber One	$2/3$ cup
Raisin Bran	$1/2$ cup
Grape Nuts	$1/4$ cup
Müeslix	$1/3$ cup
Puffed cereal	$1 1/2$ cups
Other ready-to-eat unsweetened cereals	$3/4$ cup
Sugar-coated cereals	$1/2$ cup
Shredded wheat	1 biscuit
Shredded wheat, spoon size	16 pieces

Cereals (Cooked)

Unflavored	$1/2$ cup
Flavored (add 2 fruits)	$1/2$ cup
Instant single serving packet (add $1/2$ grain)	$1/2$ cup
Coco Wheats	$1/2$ cup

Crackers/Snacks

Flatbread, Norwegian	4
Gingersnaps	3
Graham crackers ($2 1/2$" square crackers)	3
Matzoth	$3/4$ oz.
Melba toast	5 slices
Oyster crackers	24
Popcorn, air popped, no fat added	3 cups
Pretzels, very thin twisted	4
Rice cakes	2
Ry Krisp	3 triple crackers
Saltine-type crackers	6

Dried Beans/Peas/Lentils

Baked beans	$1/4$ cup
Beans and peas such as kidney, white, split blackeye (cooked)	$1/3$ cup
Lentils, cooked	$1/3$ cup

Grains

Barley, cooked	$1/3$ cup
Buckwheat	$1/2$ cup
Bulgur, cracked wheat	$1/3$ cup
Cornmeal, dry	$2 1/2$ Tbsp.
Flour	3 Tbsp.
Grits, cooked	$1/2$ cup
Millet	$1/2$ cup
Wheat Germ	3 Tbsp.
Pasta, any type such as macaroni, spaghetti, egg noodles (cooked)	$1/2$ cup

Rice, cooked

Brown	$1/3$ cup
White	$1/2$ cup
Wild	$1/2$ cup

Miscellaneous

Angelfood cake, not iced	$^1/_{12}$ th of cake
Instant hot cocoa mix (add $^1/_2$ grain)	1 packet
Pancakes, frozen microwave	1

(For additional crackers, see the Grain + Fat group.)

Vegetables

Corn	$^1/_2$ cup
Corn, cream style	$^1/_3$ cup
Corn on cob, 6" long	1
Lima beans	$^1/_2$ cup
Peas, green (canned or frozen)	$^1/_2$ cup
Plantain	$^1/_2$ cup
Potato, baked	1 small
Squash, winter (acorn or butternut)	$^3/_4$ cup
Sweet potato, yam	$^1/_3$ cup

Food Group: Grain and Fat

(Count all foods shown as 1 grain and 1 fat.)

Arrowroot cookies	5
Biscuit, 2 $^1/_2$" across	1
Biscuit mix, dry	$^1/_4$ cup
Cereal bar, Kellogg's Smart Star (add 1 fruit)	1
Chow mein noodles	$^1/_2$ cup
Cornbread, 2" cube	1
Cornbread Twist, Pillsbury	1 $^1/_2$
Chips	
Cheetos	25 or $^3/_4$ oz.
Doritos	15
Fritos	34
Potato chips, 1 $^1/_4$ oz. bag (add 1 fat)	1 bag
Ruffles Light	17
Crackers	
American Classic, any flavor	6
Bran Thins	12
Cheese Nips or Cheez-Its	24
Club	8
Hi Ho or Ritz	6
Nabisco Chocolate Grahams	2
Ritz Bits	35
Sociables	12
Teddy Grahams	20
Townhouse	8
Triscuits	6
Waverly Wafers	6
Wheat Thins	12
Wheatsworth	7
Crescent or butterflake roll	1
Croissant, plain (add 1 fat)	1 medium
Croissant, Sara Lee	1 petite
French toast (add $^1/_2$ complete protein)	1 slice
Granola bar	1 oz.
Muffin	
Blueberry, Sara Lee Free and Light	1
(count as 1 grain + 1 fruit)	

Plain, small	1
Flavored, large (add 1 fruit)	1
Noodle/Pasta/Rice varieties	
Chow mein	1/2 cup
Ramen, cooked	1/2 cup
Noodles or rice in sauce	1/2 cup
Pasta salad (add 1/2 grain + 1 fat)	1/2 cup
Rice a Roni	1/2 cup
Pancake, 4" across	2
Popcorn, oil popped or microwave (add 1 fat)	3 cups popped
Popcorn, microwave light	4 cups popped
Popcorn, Pop Secret Singles microwave (add 1/2 grain + 2 fats)	1 bag
Popover, small	1
Potato varieties	
Au gratin	1/3 cup
Cottage fries	3 oz.
Escalloped, scalloped	1/2 cup
French fries	10 medium or 1/2 cup
Hash browns	1/3 cup or 3 oz.
Mashed	1/2 cup
Salad (add 1 fat)	1/2 cup
Shoestring (add 1 fat)	3/4 cup or 1 oz.
Tater Tots	1/2 cup
Ralston Chex Snack Mix	2/3 cup
Rice Krispie bar (add 1 grain)	1/24 th of recipe
Shortbread, Lorna Doone	5
Stuffing, prepared	1/3 cup
Teabread, banana, cranberry, etc., thin-sliced	1 slice
Toaster pastry (add 1 fruit)	1
Vanilla wafers	6
Waffle, 4 1/2" square	1

Food Group: Vegetable

Vegetables are an important source of vitamins, minerals and fiber. They contain a moderate amount of complex carbohydrate and protein. Vegetables containing a larger amount of carbohydrate, such as potatoes, corn and green peas, are counted as grain units.

Unless otherwise indicated, 1 cup *raw* portion or 1/2 cup *cooked* portion is equal to one vegetable unit.

Artichoke (1/2 heart)	Leeks (12 medium)
Asparagus	Mixed vegetable, any variety (1/3 cup)
Bamboo shoots	Okra
Bean sprouts	Onions
Beets	Pea pods (snow peas)
Broccoli	Rhubarb
Brussels sprouts	Rutabaga
Cabbage	Sauerkraut
Carrots	Spinach
Cauliflower	Summer squash
Eggplant	Coczelle
Kohlrabi	Crookneck

Scallop
Spaghetti
Straight neck
Zucchini
String beans
  Green
  Yellow (wax)
Tomatoes, raw (1 medium)
Tomatoes, cherry (5-6)

Tomato catsup (3 Tbsp.)
Tomato juice
Tomato paste (2 Tbsp.)
Tomato puree ($^1/_4$ cup)
Tomato sauce ($^1/_3$ cup)
Turnips
Vegetable juice cocktail
Water chestnuts, canned
  (5-6 whole)

The raw foods listed below are not counted in vegetable units because their carbohydrate content is negligible. Limit your intake of these vegetables to 1 cup per day in order to enable yourself to "fill up" on specified units from the other food groups.

Alfalfa sprouts
Celery
Celery cabbage
Chicory
Chinese cabbage
Chives
Cucumbers
Endive
Escarole

Green pepper
Lettuce
Mushrooms
Parsley
Pickles, dill
Pimento
Radishes
Romaine
Watercress

Greens:
  Beet
  Chard
  Collards
  Dandelion
  Kale
  Mustard
  Turnip

In addition, if a single slice of raw onion or tomato is added at a meal or snack, it does not need to be counted as a vegetable unit.

For frozen vegetables in cheese sauce or cream sauce, count $^1/_2$ cup as 2 vegetables and 2 fat units.

For frozen vegetables in butter sauce, count $^1/_2$ cup as 1 vegetable and 1 fat unit.

Food Group: Fruit

Fruits are a source of carbohydrate, minerals and vitamins (especially A and C). Canned, dried, fresh and frozen fruits also contribute fiber to your meal plan. One unit is equal to any of the following items.

Fresh

Apple, small	1
Apricots, medium	4
Banana, large	$^1/_2$
Berries	
Blackberries	$^3/_4$ cup
Blueberries	1 cup
Cranberries	1 cup
Raspberries	1 cup
Strawberries	1 $^1/_2$ cups
Cantaloupe	
5" across	$^1/_3$
Cubed	1 cup
Cherries	12
Figs	2

Grapefruit	$^1/_2$
Grapes	
Small	$^1/_2$ cup or 15
Tokay	10
Honeydew melon	
Medium	$^1/_8$
Cubed	1 cup
Kiwi, large	1
Mango, small	$^1/_2$
Nectarine, medium	1
Orange, medium	1
Papaya	1 cup
Passionfruit, medium	3
Peach, medium	1
Pear, medium	1
Persimmon, medium	2
Pineapple	$^3/_4$ cup
Plum, medium	2
Pomegranate	$^1/_2$
Tangelo, tangerine, small	2
Ugli fruit, small	1
Watermelon, cubed	1 $^1/_2$ cups
Canned	
Juice-packed or packed in extra light syrup	$^1/_2$ cup
Sweetened, medium or heavy syrup	$^1/_3$ cup
Dried	
Apricots	7 halves
Currants	2 Tbsp.
Dates	3
Figs	2
Peach	2 halves
Pear	$^1/_2$
Prunes	3
Raisins	2 Tbsp.
Trail Mix dried fruits (add 1 complete protein)	1 oz.
Frozen	
Blackberries, unsweetened	$^2/_3$ cup
Blueberries, sweetened	$^1/_3$ cup
Blueberries, unsweetened	$^3/_4$ cup
Melon balls	1 cup
Mixed fruit, sweetened	$^1/_4$ cup
Raspberries, sweetened	$^1/_3$ cup
Strawberries, sweetened	$^1/_4$ cup
Strawberries, unsweetened	1 cup
Juices	
Apple	$^1/_2$ cup
Apricot nectar	$^1/_2$ cup
Apple cider	$^1/_2$ cup
Cranapricot	$^1/_3$ cup
Cranberry juice cocktail	$^1/_3$ cup
Crangrape	$^1/_3$ cup
Cranraspberry	$^1/_3$ cup
Gatorade	1 $^1/_2$ cups
Grape	$^1/_3$ cup

Grapefruit	¹/₂ cup
Guava-passionfruit	¹/₃ cup
Low calorie cranberry juice	1 ¹/₂ cups
Low calorie cranberry juice combinations	1 ¹/₂ cups
Orange	¹/₂ cup
Peach nectar	¹/₂ cup
Pear nectar	¹/₂ cup
Pineapple	¹/₂ cup

Miscellaneous

Chewy Fruit Bars	1 bar
Cranberry sauce	¹/₄ cup
Fruit Roll-ups	1 roll
Fruit Wrinkles (add ¹/₂ fruit)	1 pouch
Fun Fruits, SunKist (add ¹/₂ fruit)	1 pouch
Snack Pack Raisins, Dole (add 2 fruits)	1–1 ¹/₂ oz. box
Yogurt Raisins, Del Monte (add 1 fat)	1 pouch

Food Group: Skim Milk

Dairy foods are the primary source of calcium. There is increasing emphasis on the importance of adequate calcium intake for women throughout the premenopausal years in order to lower the risk of osteoporosis occurring later in life. Current recommendations of 800 milligrams or more of calcium per day indicate that women need at least two calcium-rich food units a day. A supplementary list of various high calcium foods and their calcium content is provided in your materials.

Milk also provides other minerals, vitamins, high quality protein and lactose (a special type of carbohydrate that enhances calcium absorption).

One unit is equal to any of the following items.

Skim or 1% milk	1 cup
Powdered non-fat dry (before adding liquid)	¹/₃ cup
Buttermilk made from skim milk	1 cup
Canned evaporated skim milk	¹/₂ cup
Yogurt made with skim milk	
Dannon Light, fruit-flavored (add ¹/₂ fruit)	1 cup
Weight Watcher's, fruit-flavored (add 1 fruit)	1 cup
Weight Watcher's, plain or Ultimate 90	1 cup
Yoplait Light, fruit-flavored	6 oz. container

(Count these as 1 milk + 1 fat unit:)

2% milk	1 cup
Canned low-fat evaporated milk	¹/₂ cup
Yogurt, low fat	
Cass Clay, fruit-flavored (add 2 fruits)	1 cup
Dannon, Fruit at the Bottom (add 2 fruits)	1 cup
Dannon, plain	1 cup
Dannon, coffee, lemon or vanilla (add 1 fruit)	1 cup
Yoplait, Custard Style, fruit-flavored (add 1 fruit)	6 oz. container
Yoplait, Original, fruit-flavored (add 1 fruit)	6 oz. container
Yoplait, Plain Original	6 oz. container

Count these foods as 1 milk + 2 fat units.

Whole milk	1 cup
Canned evaporated whole milk	¹/₂ cup

Buttermilk from whole milk	1/2 cup
Soymilk	3/4 cup
Miscellaneous	
Carnation Instant Breakfast (count as 1 milk + 1 fruit)	1 envelope
Regular cocoa mix (count as 1/2 milk + 1 fruit)	1 envelope or 2 1/2 Tbsp. dry mix
Sugar-free cocoa mix (count as 1/2 milk)	1 envelope or 2 1/2 Tbsp. dry mix

Food Group: 2% Milk

Dairy foods are the primary source of calcium. There is increasing emphasis on the importance of adequate calcium intake for women throughout the premenopausal years in order to lower the risk of osteoporosis occurring later in life. Current recommendations of 800 milligrams or more of calcium per day indicate that women need at least two calcium-rich food units a day. A supplementary list of various high calcium foods and their calcium content is provided in your materials.

Milk also provides other minerals, vitamins, high quality protein and lactose (a special type of carbohydrate that enhances calcium absorption).

One unit is equal to any of the following items.

2% milk	1 cup
Canned evaporated milk (low fat)	1/2 cup
Yogurt	
Cass Clay, fruit-flavored (add 2 fruits)	1 cup
Dannon, Fruit at the Bottom (add 2 fruits)	1 cup
Dannon, plain	1 cup
Dannon, coffee, lemon or vanilla (add 1 fruit)	1 cup
Yoplait, Custard Style or Original, fruit flavored (add 1 fruit)	6 oz. container
Yoplait, Plain Original	6 oz. container
(Count these foods as 1 milk + 1 fat unit:)	
Whole milk	1 cup
Canned evaporated whole milk	1/2 cup
Buttermilk from whole milk	1 cup
Soymilk	3/4 cup
(For any one of these foods chosen, eat one additional fat unit above the recommended number of fat units for the day:)	
Skim or 1% milk	1 cup
Powdered non-fat dry milk (before adding liquid)	1/3 cup
Buttermilk made from skim milk	1 cup
Canned evaporated skim milk	1/2 cup
Yogurt made with skim milk	
Dannon Light, fruit-flavored (add 1/2 fruit)	1 cup
Weight Watcher's, fruit-flavored (add 1 fruit)	1 cup
Weight Watcher's, plain or Ultimate 90	1 cup
Yoplait Light, fruit-flavored	6 oz. container
Carnation Instant Breakfast (count as 1 milk + 1 fruit)	1 envelope
Regular cocoa mix (count as 1/2 milk + 1 fruit)	1 envelope or 2 1/2 Tbsp. dry mix
Sugar-free cocoa mix (count as 1/2 milk)	1 envelope or 2 1/2 Tbsp. dry mix

B. Expanded Food Groups

Food Group: Sweets

Foods listed below contain carbohydrate. Although they do not contribute significant amounts of other nutrients, these can add variety to your meal plan when used in moderation. Because these foods and fruit supply similar amounts of carbohydrate in amounts shown, one unit from the sweets group may be counted as one unit of fruit. The majority of fruit units recommended on your meal plan should be chosen as fruit — not sweets.

Beverages
Imitation fruit drink (KoolAid, Tang, Hi-C, etc.)	½ cup
Lemonade	½ cup
Regular soft drinks	½ cup

Candy and Gum
Caramels	½ oz. or 2
Gum, regular	3 sticks
Gumdrops	1 oz. or 4
Hard candy (sour balls, butterscotch pieces, etc.)	½ oz. or 3
Jelly beans	¾ oz. or 8
Licorice	½ oz. or 2 Nibs
Lifesavers	8
Marshmallows	3 large

Condiments
Honey	1 Tbsp.
Jam, jelly, marmalade	1 Tbsp.
Molasses	1 Tbsp.
Pancake syrup	1 Tbsp.
Pancake syrup, light	2 Tbsp.
Sugar, brown (packed)	1 Tbsp.
Sugar, granulated	1 Tbsp.
Sugar, powdered	4 tsp.
Syrup (chocolate, strawberry, caramel, butterscotch, etc.)	1 Tbsp.

Miscellaneous
Barbecue sauce	2 Tbsp.
Jello, flavored, with sugar	⅓ cup
Jello 1-2-3 Gelatin With Two Toppings (add 1 fruit)	⅔ cup
Jello Gelatin Pops	2
Popsicle	1 twin bar

Food Group: Desserts

Foods found in this group provide primarily carbohydrate and fat. Some of the milk-based desserts are good sources of calcium, providing 140 milligrams or more of calcium per serving. These desserts are shown by an asterisk.

Your maintenance meal plan does allow for inclusion of desserts in moderation. The reason: The other food groups included in your meal plan deliver desirable amounts of complex carbohydrate, protein, fat, fiber, vitamins and minerals to meet your nutritional needs. There remains room for a dessert option to help you reach your maintenance energy needs. Remember: no one food is fattening when consumed in moderate proportion to your energy needs.

When a unit is shown as a fraction, this indicates a fraction of the entire product prepared according to directions.

	Grain	Fat	Fruit	Skim Milk
Cakes				
Angelfood or sponge cake, glazed, 1/12	2		1	
Bundt cake from mix, 1/16	1	2	1 1/2	
Carrot cake, Sara Lee Lights	1	1		
Cheesecake, Jello No Bake, 1/10	1	2	1	
Cheesecake, Royal Lite, 1/6	1	1	1	
Cheesecake, Sara Lee Classic, 1 cheesecake	1	3		
Cheesecake, Sara Lee Light Classics,	1	1	1	
Coffeecake, Sara Lee, 1/8	1	2	1	
Commercial cake mix, unfrosted 1/12	2	2		
Commercial cake mix, "light", unfrosted, 1/12 DeLights, Lovin' Lites, Supermoist Light	1	1	1	
Cupcake, iced, homemade or Hostess, 1	1	1	1	
Frosting/icing from mix, 2 Tbsp.		1/2	1	
MicroRave Cake Mix with Frosting, 1/8	1	2	1	
Pound cake, plain, 1/12	1	2	1	
Pound cake, Sara Lee Free and Light, 1 slice	1			
Twinkie, Hostess, 1	1	1	1	
Candy Bars				
Almond Joy, 1.76 oz. bar	1	3	1	
Hershey Kisses, 8	1	2	1	
Hershey plain milk chocolate, 1.65 oz. bar	1	3	1	
Kit Kat, 1.625 oz. bar	1	3	1	
M & M's, plain, 1.59 oz. package	1	2	1	
Milky Way, 2.24 oz. bar	1	2	2	
Reese's Peanut Butter Cups, 1.8 oz. package	1	3	1	
Snickers, 2.16 oz. bar	1	3	1	
Three Musketeers, 2.3 oz. bar	1	2	2	
Cookies				
Animal Crackers, 15	1	1	1	
Brownie, unfrosted, 2" × 2" × 1", 1	1	2	1	
Duncan Hines Specialty Mix Cookie, 1/22	1	2	1	
Homemade 3" diameter, 2	1	2	1	
MicroRave Frosted Brownie, 1/8	1	2	1	
Oreo Big Stuf, 1	1	2	1	
Oreo Double Stuf, 3	1	2	1	
Sandwich cookie, 1 1/2" diameter, 2	1	1		
Cream puff, frosted with filling, 1	1	4		1
Crisp or cobbler, fruit, 1/2 cup	1	1	1	
Custard, any variety, 1/2 cup*		1		1
Doughnuts				
Cake, plain, 1	1	1		
Cake, frosted, 1	1	2	1	
Raised, 1	1	1		
Eclair, frosted with filling, 1	1	2	1	
Frozen				
Bon Bon Ice Cream Nuggets, 6	1	2	1	
Cookies 'n Cream Sandwich, Oreo, 1	1	2		
Eskimo Pie, sugar-free, 1		1	1/2	
Frozen yogurt, any flavor, 3/4 cup	1		1	

	Grain	Fat	Fruit	Skim Milk
Fruit ice, sherbet, sorbet, 1/2 cup			2	
Ice cream, any flavor, 1/2 cup	1	2		
Ice cream, Haagen-Dazs, any flavor, 1/2 cup	1	3	1/2	
Ice cream bar, Dove or Haagen-Dazs, 1	1	4	1	
Ice cream bar	1	2		
Ice cream bar, Three Musketeers, 2 oz.		2	1	
Ice cream sandwich, 1	2	1		
Ice cream snack bar, Three Musketeers, 3/4 oz.		1	1/2	
Ice milk, soft serve ice milk, 1/2 cup	1	1		
Milkshake, thick, 1 cup*	3	3	1	
Pudding Pop, 2	2	1		
Simple Pleasures Frozen Dairy Dessert, any flavor, 1/2 cup	1 1/2			
Sealtest (Knudsen) Free Nonfat Frozen Dessert, 1/2 cup	1		1/2	
Pie				
Cherry Streusel, Sara Lee Free and Light	1/2		2	
Fruit type, double crust, 9" diameter, 1/8	1	2	2	
Cream type, single crust, 9" diameter, 1/8	2	3		
Snack pie, Hostess, fruit flavor, 1	2	4	1	
Pudding				
Regular bread pudding, 1/2 cup	2	1	1/2	
Regular, made with 2% or whole milk, 1/2 cup	1	1	1	
Sugar-free NutraSweet with skim milk, 1/2 cup	1			
Tapioca, 1/2 cup	1	1	1	
Studel, Pillsbury Toaster, 1	1	2	1	
Sweet roll, Apple Danish, Sara Lee Free and Light	1		1	
Sweet roll, Pillsbury cinnamon from refrigerator dough, 2	1	2	1	
Turnover, Pillsbury, 1	1/2	2	1	

Food Group: Free Foods

(The following foods may be used as desired.)

Beverages
- Carbonated beverages, sugar-free
- Carbonated water
- Club soda
- Coffee
- Decaffeinated coffee, tea
- Herbal tea
- Soft drink mixes, sugar-free
- Tea, hot or iced, sugar-free
- Tonic water, sugar-free

Condiments and Seasonings
- Butter Buds, Molly McButter
- Herbs
- Horseradish
- Soy sauce
- Spices
- Tabasco sauce
- Worcestershire sauce

Miscellaneous

- Artificial sweetener
- Gelatin, unflavored, plain
- Hard candy, sugar-free
- Nonstick pan spray

The following foods have a very small caloric content in the amounts shown. If you customarily include more than three servings of these foods per day, your dietitian will discuss how to count them in your meal plan.

Bacon flavor bits	1 tsp.
Catsup	1 Tbsp.
Chewing gum, sugar-free	3 sticks
Chili sauce	1 Tbsp.
Crystal Light Bars	1 bar
Cocoa, unsweetened	1 Tbsp.
Cranberries, unsweetened	1/2 cup
Dill pickle	1 medium
Gelatin, sugar-free, flavored	1/2 cup
Jam/Jelly, sugar-free	2 Tbsp.
Low calorie (nonfat) salad dressing such as Hidden Valley Ranch Take Heart Dressings	2 Tbsp.
Mustard	2 Tbsp.
Pancake syrup, sugar-free	2 Tbsp.
Reduced calorie jellies or preserves	1 tsp.
Rhubarb, unsweetened	1/2 cup
Steak sauce	1 Tbsp.
Sweet pickle	1 small
Sweet pickle relish	1 Tbsp.
Taco sauce	3 Tbsp.

As stated in the Vegetable group, page 20, limit your intake of the specified salad greens to 1 cup per day. Excessive intake of these greens may prevent you from consuming adequate calories and nutrients from other foods.

Food Group: Combination Foods

Included below are common examples of combination foods such as casseroles and soups. Refer to the International food groups for combinations such as chow mein, lasagna and tacos.

	Complete Protein Subgroup 2	Grain	Fat	Veg	Fruit
Breaded chicken products					
Banquet:					
Chicken Nuggets, 3 oz.	1	1	2		
Breaded Chicken patty, 3 oz.	1	1	2		
Breaded Chicken Sticks, 3 oz.	1	1	2		
Tyson:					
Chick'n Quick Breast Patty, 3 oz.	2	1/2	2		
Chick'n Chunks, 6 pieces	1	1	2		
Chick'n Sticks, 3 sticks	1	1	2		
Chicken Corn Dog, 1	1	2	2		
Breaded Fish Products					
Gorton's Crispy Batter Dipped Fish Fillet, 1	1	1	2		

	Complete Protein Subgroup 2	Grain	Fat	Veg	Fruit
Mrs. Pauls:					
Fish cakes, 2 cakes	1	2	2		
Crispy Crunchy Fish Sticks, 4	1	1	2		
Fried Shrimp, 3 oz.	1	1	1		
Light Breaded Fish Fillet, 1	2	1 1/2			
Van De Kamp's Fish Nuggets, 2 oz.	1	1/2	1		
Casseroles, any variety, 1 cup	2	2	1		
Convenience combination snacks/meals					
Campbells Souper Combo					
Chicken Noodle O's Soup	1	2	2		
Chili With Beans and Hot Dog on a Bun	2	3	2		
Tomato Soup and Grilled Cheese Sandwich	2	2	2		
Vegetable Soup and Cheeseburger	2	2	2		
Light Balance					
Beef Americana (subgroup1)	1	2			
Beef and Pasta Bordeaux (subgroup 1)	1	2			
Chicken Fiesta (subgroup 1)	1	2			
Mushroom Stroganoff		2	1		
Pasta and Garden Vegetables		2		1	
Louis Rich Lunch Breaks					
Oven Roasted Turkey Breast and Cheddar	3	1 1/2	2		
Smoked Turkey and Monterey Jack	3	1 1/2	2		
Turkey Ham and Swiss	3	1 1/2	1		
Turkey Salami and Cheddar	3	1 1/2	3		
Lunch Bucket					
Chicken Noodle Soup		1	1		
Lasagna		3	1		
Spaghetti 'n meat sauce		3	2		
Oscar Mayer Lunchables					
Ham and Swiss	2	1	2	1	
Turkey and Cheddar	2	1	1	1	
Oscar Mayer Lunchables Deluxe					
Ham and Roast Beef	3	1 1/2	2		
Turkey and Ham	3	1 1/2	1		
Oscar Mayer Zappetites					
Deluxe Italian Bread Pizza	1	1	2		
Ham and Cheese Stuffed Sandwich	1	1	2		
Italian Bread Sausage Pizza	1	1	2		
Mexican Stuffed Sandwich	1	1	2		
Sausage Biscuit	1	1	2		
Sausage, Egg and Cheese Biscuit	1	1	2		
Snack Cheeseburger	1	1	2		
Snack Hamburger	1	1	1		
Snack Chili Cheese Dog	1	1	1		
Stuffed Potato Skin		1	2		
Western Omelet Stuffed Sandwich		1	2		
Corned beef hash, 1 cup	2	2			
French toast, 2 slices	1	2	1		
Macaroni and cheese mix, 1 cup prepared	1	2	2		
Quiche Lorraine, 1/8 of 9" pie	1	1/2	5		

	Complete Protein Subgroup 2	Grain	Fat	Veg	Fruit
Sandwiches					
(egg salad, chicken salad, ham salad or tuna salad)	1	2	3		
¹/₃ cup salad mixture + 2 slices of unbuttered bread					
Sausage biscuits, Jimmy Dean, 1		2	3		
Sloppy Joe					
¹/₆ th serving of 1-15¹/₂ oz. can Manwich Sauce +	2	3			
1 pound lean ground beef + unbuttered bun					
Soups					
Bean, 1 cup	1	1			
Bouillon (free food)	—	—	—	—	
Chunky, any variety, 1-10³/₄ can	1	1		1	
Cream, made with water, 1 cup		1	1		
Vegetable or broth-based, 1 cup		1			
Stew, meat and vegetable, 1 cup	2	2			
Stuffed green pepper, 1 average	2	2			

Food Group: International

	Complete Protein Subgroup 2	Grain	Fat	Veg.
ITALIAN				
Canned pasta or spaghetti meals				
Spaghettios/spaghetti with meatballs (1 cup)	1	1¹/₂	1	
Ragu pasta meals, ¹/₂ of 15 oz. jar	1	1¹/₂		
Lasagna, 3" square	3	2	1	1
Mannicotti, 6", 1 filled	2	2	1	
Pizza				
French bread type, ¹/₂ pkg.	1	3	2	
Frozen or refrigerated				
14-16 oz., ¹/₆	1	1	1	
22-24 oz., ¹/₆	1	2	1	
Tombstone Light, 19-22 oz., ¹/₅	1	2	1	
(See "Food Group: Restaurants" for Pizza Hut information)				
Microwave pizza				
Pillsbury, ¹/₂	1	2	2	
Tony's, ¹/₂	1	2¹/₂	3	
Ratatouilli, ¹/₂ cup		2	1	
Ravioli, 1 cup	1	2	1	1
Spaghetti sauce				
Commercial, without meat or meat-flavored, ¹/₂ cup		1	1	
Commercial, with meat added, ³/₄ cup	1	1	1	
Veal parmesan (breaded cutlet with cheese and sauce),	4	1		
4 oz. cutlet				
MEXICAN				
Burrito				
Beef, 6" tortilla	2	2	1	
Bean, 6" tortilla	1	3	1	
Frozen, any variety	1	2	1	
Chili with beans, 1 cup	2	2	2	
Chili rellenos, 7"	2	2	2	
Enchilada, 6" tortilla made with meat or cheese	2	2	1	

	Complete Protein Subgroup 2	Grain	Fat	Veg.
Gaucamole, 2 Tbsp.			1	
Hot sauce or taco sauce, 1 Tbsp. (free food)	—	—	—	—
Refried beans, 1/3 cup		1	2	
Spanish rice, 1/2 cup		1	1	
Taco, 1		2	1	1
Taco shell, 6" diameter		1		
Tortilla				
Small, 6" diameter		1		
Large, 12" diameter		2		
Tostada				
With refried beans		2	1	
With meat	1	1	1	

ORIENTAL

	Complete Protein Subgroup 2	Grain	Fat	Veg.
Chow mein without noodles or rice, 2 cups	2	2		1
Chop suey without noodles or rice, 2 cups	3	1		1
Egg foo young, 1 cup	2		2	1
Egg foo young sauce, 1/2 cup				1
Egg roll, 1	1	1	1	1
Fortune cookie, 2		1		
Fried rice, no meat, 1/2 cup		1	2	
Fried rice, with meat and egg, 1 cup	1	1	1	1
Noodles				
Chow mein, 1/2 cup		1	1	
Egg, 1/2 cup		1		
Pepper steak, 1 cup	3	1		1
Soy sauce, 1 Tbsp. (free food)	—	—	—	—
Sweet and sour pork, 1 cup	2	2	2	
Won tons, fried, 4		1	4	
Won ton soup (2 won tons in broth)		1	1	

Food Group: Frozen Entrees, Meals

Selected products have been included from various companies that produce frozen main courses and meals.

	Complete Protein Subgroup 1	Grain	Fat	Veg.	Fruit
HEALTHY CHOICE DINNERS					
Beef Enchilada, 12 3/4 oz.	1	3			1
Chicken Dijon, 11 oz.	2	2		1	
Chicken Enchilada, 12 3/4 oz.		4	1		
Herb Roasted Chicken, 12 1/3 oz.	2	2		1	
Mesquite Chicken, 10 1/2 oz.	2	4			
Pasta Primavera, 11 oz.		3 1/2	1		
Salisbury Steak, 11 1/2 oz.	1	3	1		
Salsa Chicken, 11 1/4 oz.	2	2		1	
Shrimp Marinara, 10 1/2 oz.		3		1	
Yankee Pot Roast, 11 oz.	2	2 1/2			
HEALTHY CHOICE ENTREES					

	Complete Protein Subgroup 1	Grain	Fat	Veg.	Fruit
Baked Cheese Ravioli, 9 oz.	1	2		1	
Beef Fajitas, 7 oz.	2	2			
Beef Pepper Steak, 9 1/2 oz.	1	2		1	
Cheese Mannicotti, 9 1/4 oz.	1	2		1	
Chicken A' L'Orange, 9 oz.	1	2		1	
Chicken and Vegetables, 11 1/2 oz.	2	2			
Chicken Chow Mein, 8 1/2 oz.	2	2			
Chicken Fajitas, 7 oz.	1	2			
Chicken Fettucini, 8 1/2 oz.	2	2			
Fettucini Alfredo, 8 oz.		2	1	1	
Glazed Chicken, 8 1/2 oz.	2	2			
Lasagna with Meat Sauce, 10 oz.	2	2		1	
Linguini with Shrimp, 9 1/2 oz.	1	2 1/2			
Mandarin Chicken, 11 oz.	2	2		1	
Rigatoni in Meat Sauce, 9 1/2 oz.	1	2		1	
Seafood Newburg, 8 oz.	1	2			
Roasted Turkey and Mushrooms in Gravy, 8 1/2 oz.	2	1 1/2			
Sole with Lemon Butter Sauce, 8 1/4 oz.	1	2		1	
Spaghetti with Meat Sauce, 10 oz.	1	3			
Zucchini Lasagna, 11 1/2 oz.	1	2		1	
STOUFFERS RIGHT CHOICE					
Beef Dijon with Pasta and Vegetables, 9 1/2 oz.	2	2	1		
Beef Ragout with Rice Pilaf 10 oz.	2	2		1	
Chicken Tenderloins in Barbecue Sauce with Rice Pilaf, 8 3/4 oz.	2	2		1	
Chicken Tenderloins in Peanut Sauce with Linguini and Vegetables, 9 1/4 oz.	3	2			
Chicken Italiano with Fettucini and Vegetables, 9 5/8 oz.	3	2			
Fiesta Beef with Corn Pasta 8 7/8 oz.	1	2		1	
Homestyle Pot Roast, 9 1/4 oz.	2	1		1	
Sesame Chicken, 10 oz.	2	1	1	1	
Sliced Turkey in a Mild Curry Sauce with Rice Pilaf, 8 oz.	2	2 1/2	1		
Shrimp Primavera, 9 oz.	1	2	1		
Vegetarian Chili		3	1		
ARMOUR CLASSIC LITES					
Beef Pepper Steak, 11 1/4 oz.	2	2			
Beef Stroganoff, 11 1/4 oz.	2	2			
Chicken Ala King, 11 1/4 oz.	2	2		1	
Chicken Oriental, 10 oz.	2	1		1	
Shrimp Creole, 11 1/4 oz.		3		1	
Sweet and Sour Chicken, 11 oz.	1	2		1	
ARMOUR CLASSICS					
Chicken Fettucini, 11 oz.	2	2			
Chicken Mesquite, 9 1/2 oz.	1	3	2		
Chicken Parmigiana, 11 1/2 oz.	2	2	2		
Glazed Chicken, 10 3/4 oz.	2	1 1/2	2		
Meat Loaf, 11 1/4 oz.	2	2	2		
Salisbury Steak, 11 1/4 oz.	3	1 1/2	2		
Swedish Meatballs, 11 1/4 oz.	2	1 1/2	2		

	Complete Protein Subgroup 1	Grain	Fat	Veg.	Fruit
Turkey with Dressing and Gravy, 11 $^{1}/_{2}$ oz.	2	2	1	1	
BANQUET					
Beans and Frankfurters, 10 oz.		3	3		
Beef Enchilada, 11 oz.		3	2	1	
Fish Platter, 8 oz.	1	2		1	
Fried Chicken, 9 oz.	2	2	4	1	
Macaroni and Cheese, 9 oz.		2 $^{1}/_{2}$	2		
Salisbury Steak, 9 oz.	1	2	2		
Spaghetti and Meat Sauce, 8 $^{3}/_{4}$ oz.		1 $^{1}/_{2}$	1		
Turkey and Gravy with Dressing, 9 $^{1}/_{4}$ oz.	1	2	2		
LE MENU					
Beef Sirloin Tips, 11 $^{1}/_{2}$ oz.	3	2	1		
Beef Stroganoff, 10 oz.	3	2	2		
Chicken a la King, 10 $^{1}/_{4}$ oz.	2	2	1		
Chicken Gordon Bleu, 11 oz.	2	3	2		
Pepper Steak, 11 $^{1}/_{2}$ oz.	3	2	1		
Sweet and Sour Chicken, 11 $^{1}/_{4}$ oz.	1	2 $^{1}/_{2}$	2	1	
Yankee Pot Roast, 10 oz.	3	2			
STOUFFERS					
Beef Chop Suey with Rice, 12 oz.	1	2	1	1	
Beef Stroganoff with Parsley Noodles, 9 $^{3}/_{4}$ oz.	3	2	1		
Cashew Chicken in Sauce with Rice, 9 $^{1}/_{2}$ oz.	3	2			
Cheese Enchiladas, 10 $^{1}/_{8}$ oz.	2	2	6	1	
Chicken a La King with Rice, 9 $^{1}/_{2}$ oz.	2	2 $^{1}/_{2}$			
Chicken Chow Mein without Noodles, 8 oz.	1			2	
Chicken Divan, 8 $^{1}/_{2}$ oz.	3	1	1		
Creamed Chicken, 6 $^{1}/_{2}$ oz.	2	$^{1}/_{2}$	2		
Creamed Chipped Beef, $^{1}/_{2}$ of 11 oz. pkg.	2	$^{1}/_{2}$	1		
Escalloped Chicken with Noodles, 10 oz.	2	2	3		
Green Pepper Steak with Rice, 10 $^{1}/_{2}$ oz.	2	2		1	
Ham and Asparagus Bake, 6 $^{1}/_{4}$ oz.	2	2	5		
Lasagna, 10 $^{1}/_{2}$ oz.	3	2		1	
Lobster Newburg, 6 $^{1}/_{2}$ oz.	2	$^{1}/_{2}$	4		
Macaroni and Cheese, 12 oz.	1	1 $^{1}/_{2}$	1 $^{1}/_{2}$		
Meat Pie (Beef, Chicken, or Turkey), 10 oz.	2	2	4	1	
Spaghetti with Meatballs, 12 $^{5}/_{8}$ oz.	2	3	2		
Stuffed Green Peppers w/Beef in Tomato Sauce, $^{1}/_{2}$ of 15 oz. pkg.	1	1	1	1	
Tuna Noodle Casserole, 10 oz.	2	2	2		
Turkey Tetrazzini, 10 oz.	2	2	2		
Vegetable Lasagna, 10 $^{1}/_{2}$ oz.	2	2	3		
STOUFFERS LEAN CUISINE					
Cheese Cannelloni with Tomato Sauce, 9 $^{1}/_{8}$ oz.	2	1 $^{1}/_{2}$		1	
Chicken Chow Mein with Rice, 9 oz.	1	2		1	
Fillet of Fish Florentine, 9 $^{5}/_{8}$ oz. (Subgroup 1)	3	1			
Glazed Chicken with Vegetable Rice, 8 $^{1}/_{2}$ oz. (Subgroup 1)	3	1		1	
Oriental Beef with Vegetables and Rice, 8 $^{5}/_{8}$ oz.	2	2			
Spaghetti with Beef Sauce, 11 $^{1}/_{2}$ oz.	1	3			
Stuffed Cabbage with Meat in Tomato Sauce, 10 $^{3}/_{4}$ oz.	2	1		1	

	Complete Protein Subgroup 1	Grain	Fat	Veg	Fruit
Turkey Dijon, 9 1/2 oz.	2	1 1/2			
SWANSON					
Barbecue Flavored Fried Chicken, 10 oz.	2	3	2		1
Fish 'n Chips, 10 oz.	3	4	1		
Macaroni and Cheese, 12 1/4 oz.	1	3	2		
Spaghetti and Meatballs, 12 1/2 oz.	1	3	2		
Turkey Dinner, 11 1/2 oz.	2	3		1	
Meat Pie					
Beef, 7 oz.	1	2	3	1	
Chicken, 7 oz.	1	2	3	1	

Food Group: Restaurant Foods

	Complete Protein Subgroup 2	Grain	Fat	Veg.	Fruit
BURGER KING					
Sandwiches/Entrees:					
Bacon Double Cheeseburger	4	2	2		
Bacon Double Cheeseburger Deluxe	4	2	4		
BK Broiler Chicken Sandwich	3	2	1		
Burger Buddies	2	2	1		
Cheeseburger	2	2	1		
Cheeseburger Deluxe	2	2	3		
Chicken Sandwich	2	4	6		
Chicken Tenders, 6 pieces	2	1	1		
Chicken/Fish Tenders Dipping Sauces					
Barbecue					1
Honey					1
Ranch			4		
Sweet and Sour					1
Tartar			4		
Double Cheeseburger	3	2	3		
Double Whopper	5	3	6		
Double Whopper with Cheese	6	3	6		
Fish Tenders	1	1	2		
Hamburger	1	2	1		
Hamburger Deluxe	1	2	3		
Mushroom Swiss Double Cheeseburger	4	2	1		
Ocean Catch Fish Filet	2	3	3		
Whopper	3	3	4		
Whopper with Cheese	3	3	6		
Whopper Jr.	1	2	2		
Whopper Jr. with Cheese	2	2	2		
Salads/Dressings					
Chef Salad	2	1/2			
Chunky Chicken Salad (Subgroup 1)	3	1/2			
Garden Salad	1	1/2			
Side Salad		1/2			
Bleu Cheese Dressing, 1/2 pkg.			3		
French Dressing, 1/2 pkg.		1/2	2		
Olive Oil and Vinegar Dressing, 1/2 pkg.			3		

	Complete Protein Subgroup 2	Grain	Fat	Veg.	Fruit
Ranch Dressing, ½ pkg.			4		
Reduced Calorie Light Italian Dressing, ½ pkg.			2		
Thousand Island Dressing, ½ pkg.		½	3		
Other Items					
French Fries, Regular		1½	3		
Milkshake, Any Flavor		2	2		1
Onion Rings, Regular		2	3		
Snack Pie, Cherry or Apple		1	3		2
Breakfast					
Breakfast Croissan'wich					
Bacon, Egg, Cheese	2	1	3		
Ham, Egg, Cheese	2	1	2		
Sausage, Egg, Cheese	2	1½	6		
Scrambled Egg Platter	1	2	5		
French Toast Platter with Bacon		3	6		
French Toast Platter with Sausage	1	3	8		
Mini Muffins					
Blueberry		2	3		½
Lemon Poppyseed		1	4		1
Raisin Oat		2	2		1

DAIRY QUEEN
Sandwiches/Entrees

	Complete Protein Subgroup 2	Grain	Fat	Veg.	Fruit
Chicken Fillet Sandwich, Breaded	2	2	2	1	
Chicken Fillet Sandwich, Grilled	2	2		1	
Fish Fillet Sandwich	1	2	2	1	
Fish Fillet Sandwich with Cheese	2	2	2	1	
Hamburgers					
Single	2	2	1		
Double	4	2	1		
Single with Cheese	2	2	2		
Double with Cheese	4	2	3		
DQ Homestyle Ultimate	5	2	4		
Hot Dogs					
Regular	1	2	2		
With Chili	1	1½	3		
With Cheese	1	1½	3		
Super	2	3	6		
Salads/Dressings					
Garden Salad		½		1	
Side Salad				1	
Dressings					
French Reduced Calorie, ½ pkg.			1		
Thousand Island, ½ pkg.			2		

	Complete Protein Subgroup 2	Grain	Fat	Fruit	Skim Milk
Other Items					
Banana Split			3	2	3
Blizzard					

	Complete Protein Subgroup 2	Grain	Fat	Fruit	Skim Milk
Small, Heath, 12 oz.		2	5	3	1/2
Regular, Heath, 16 oz.		4	7	3	1/2
Large, Heath, 21 oz.		5	9	5	1/2
Small, Strawberry, 12 oz.		2	2	2	1/2
Regular, Strawberry, 16 oz.		3 1/2	3	2	1/2
Large, Strawberry, 21 oz.		3 1/2	4	4	1/2
Breeze					
Small, Heath, 12 oz.		2	2	3	1/2
Regular, Heath, 16 oz.		4	4	3	1/2
Small, Strawberry, 12 oz.		2		2	1/2
Regular, Strawberry, 16 oz.		2 1/2		3	1/2
Buster Bar		2	6	1	
Cones					
Small		1 1/2	1		
Regular		2	1	1	
Large		2	2	1	1/2
Small, Dipped		1	2	1	
Regular, Dipped		2	3	1	
Large, Dipped		2	5	2	
Regular, Yogurt		1 1/2		1	
Large, Yogurt		2 1/2		1	
Queen's Choice, Big Scoop		1	3	2	
Cups					
Regular, Yogurt		2 1/2			
Large, Yogurt		2 1/2		1	
Dilly Bar		1 1/2	2		
DQ Sandwich		1 1/2	1		
French Fries, Small		2	2		
French Fries, Regular		2 1/2	3		
Hot Fudge Brownie Delight		4	6	3	
Malt — Terms used for sizes vary; see ounces					
16 oz.		2	3	4	1
21 oz.		4	4	5	1/2
32 oz.		8	6	5	1
Mr. Misty — Terms used for sizes vary; see ounces					
16 oz.				4	
21 oz.				5	
32 oz.				8	
Onion Rings, Regular		2	2		
Peanut Buster Parfait		4	7	2	1/2
Shake — Terms used for sizes vary; see ounces					
16 oz.		2	3	3	1
21 oz.		2	3	4	1
32 oz.		4	5	5	1
Sundae, Waffle Cone		2	2	2	

	Complete Protein Subgroup 2	Grain	Fat	Veg.	Fruit
HARDEE'S					
Sandwiches/Entrees					
Bacon Cheeseburger	4	2	4		

	Complete Protein Subgroup 2	Grain	Fat	Veg.	Fruit
Big Deluxe	3	2	3		
Big Roast Beef	2	2			
Big Twin	2	2	3		
Cheeseburger	2	2	1		
Chicken Fillet Sandwich	2	3	1		
Chicken Stix, 6 piece	2	1			
Fisherman's Fillet Sandwich	2	3	3		
Grilled Chicken Sandwich (subgroup 1)	3	2			
Hamburger	1	2	1		
Hot Dog	1	2	2		
Hot Ham and Cheese	2	2			
Mushroom 'N' Swiss Burger	3	2	2		
Quarter Pound Cheeseburger	3	2	3		
Roast Beef Sandwich, regular	1	2	1		
Real Lean Deluxe	2	2		1	
Turkey Club	3	2			
Salads/Dressings					
Chef Salad (Subgroup 1)	3	¹/₂			
Chicken 'N' Pasta Salad	3	1¹/₂			
Garden Salad	2		1		
Side Salad (free food)	—	—	—		
Other Items					
Apple Turnover		1	2		
Big Cookie		1	3		
Cool Twist Cone, any flavor		1	1		
French Fries					
Crispy Curls		2¹/₂	3		
Regular		2	2		
Large		3	3		
Milkshake, vanilla		3	2		1
Milkshake, chocolate or strawberry		3	2		3
Breakfast					
Bacon and Egg Biscuit	1	2¹/₂	4		
Canadian Rise 'N' Shine Biscuit	2	2¹/₂	3		
Country Ham Biscuit	1	2	2		
Country Ham and Egg Biscuit	1	2¹/₂	3		
Sausage Biscuit	1	2	5		
Sausage and Egg Biscuit	2	2¹/₂	4		
Steak Biscuit	1	3	5		
Steak and Egg Biscuit	2	3	4		

KENTUCKY FRIED CHICKEN
Sandwiches/Entrees
Chicken

	Complete Protein Subgroup 2	Grain	Fat	Veg.	Fruit
Extra Tasty Crispy					
Center Breast	4	1			
Side Breast	3	1	1		
Drumstick	2	¹/₂	1		
Thigh	2	1	4		
Wing	2	¹/₂	2		
Original Recipe					
Center Breast (Subgroup 1)	4	¹/₂			

	Complete Protein Subgroup 2	Grain	Fat	Veg.	Fruit
Side Breast	2	1	1		
Drumstick	2	1/2			
Thigh	2	1/2	2		
Wing	2	1/2			
Chicken Littles Sandwich	1	1	1		
Colonel's Chicken Sandwich	2	2 1/2	3		
Hot Wings	3	1	2		
Kentucky Nuggets, 6 piece	2	1	1		
Other Items					
Buttermilk Biscuit		2	2		
Mashed Potatoes and Gravy		1	1/2		
Cole Slaw		1	1		
Corn on the Cob		2	1		
French Fries		2	2		
Kentucky Nugget Sauces					
Barbecue					1/2
Honey					1
Mustard					1/2
Sweet and Sour					1
Potato Salad		1	2		
Kentucky Fries		2	3		

MCDONALD'S
Sandwiches/Entrees

	Complete Protein Subgroup 2	Grain	Fat	Veg.	Fruit
Big Mac	3	3	2		
Cheeseburger	1	2	2		
Chicken Fajita, 1	1	1	1	1	
Filet-O-Fish	1	2 1/2	2		
Hamburger	1	2	1		
McLean Deluxe	2	2		1	
McChicken	2	2 1/2	2		
McDLT	3	2	4	1	
Quarter Pounder	3	2	1		
Quarter Pounder with Cheese	3	2	3		
Chicken McNuggets, 6 pieces	2	1	1		
Chicken McNugget Sauce, 1 packet					
Barbecue					1
Honey					1
Hot Mustard		1/2	1		
Sweet and Sour					1
Salads/Dressings					
Chef Salad	2		1		
Chunky Chicken Salad (Subgroup 1)	3		1		
Garden Salad			1		
Side Salad			1		
Bacon Bits (free food)	—	—	—	—	—
Croutons		1/2			
Dressings					
Bleu Cheese, 1/2 pkg.			3		
French, 1/2 pkg.			2	1	
Lite Vinaigrette, 1/2 pkg. (free food)		—	—	—	—

	Complete Protein Subgroup 2	Grain	Fat	Veg.	Fruit
Ranch, ½ pkg.			3		
Red French Reduced Calorie, ½ pkg.			1		½
Thousand Island, ½ pkg.			3		½
Other Items					
Cookies					
McDonaldland		2	2		
Chocolaty Chip		2	3	1	
French Fries, Regular		2	2		
French Fries, Large		3	3		
Frozen Yogurt Cone, Vanilla		1½			
Frozen Yogurt Sundae with Hot Fudge		2	1		1½
Skim Milk					
Milkshake, any flavor		4			
Snack Pie, apple or cherry		1	3		1
Breakfast					
Apple Bran Muffin		2			1
Biscuits					
Biscuit with Biscuit Spread		2	3		
Biscuit w/Bacon, Egg and Cheese	2	2	3		
Biscuit with Sausage	1	2	5		
Biscuit with Sausage and Egg	2	2	5		
Breakfast Burrito	1	1	2	1	
Danish, apple or iced cheese		3	4		
English Muffin with Butter		2	1		
Hashbrown Potatoes		1	1		
Hotcakes with Butter and Syrup		3	2		2
McMuffin					
Egg McMuffin	2	2			
Sausage McMuffin	2	2	2		
Sausage McMuffin with Egg	2	2	3		
Pork Sausage	1		2		
Scrambled Eggs	2				
PIZZA HUT					
Hand-tossed Pizza, 1 slice of medium pizza					
Cheese	2	2			
Pepperoni	1	2	1		
Supreme	1	2	1		
Super Supreme	1	2	2		
Pan Pizza, 1 slice of medium pizza					
Cheese	1	2	1		
Pepperoni	1	2	1		
Supreme	1	2	2		
Super Supreme	1	2	2		
Thin 'n Crispy Pizza, 1 slice of medium pizza					
Cheese	1	1	1	1	
Pepperoni	1	1	1	1	
Supreme	1	1	1	1	
Super Supreme	1	1	1	1	
Personal Pan Pizza					
Pepperoni, 1 whole pizza	3	5	3		
Supreme, 1 whole pizza	3	5	3		

	Complete Protein Subgroup 2	Grain	Fat	Veg.	Fruit

RED LOBSTER

Entrees ordered from the dinner (supper) menu
Subgroup 1

	Complete Protein Subgroup 2	Grain	Fat	Veg.	Fruit
Alaskan Snow Crab Legs	9				
Norwegian Salmon, broiled	7			1	
Rock Lobster Tail, broiled	7				
Shrimp, grilled, 2 skewers	7				
Swordfish, broiled	5				
Walleye Pike, broiled	7				

(The lunch portion of most entrees is approximately half as large as the dinner portion.)

Accompaniments to the entrees listed above

	Complete Protein Subgroup 2	Grain	Fat	Veg.	Fruit
Coleslaw			1	1	
Garlic Bread		1	1		
Hush Puppies, 2		1/2	1		
Rice Pilaf (1-1 1/4 cups)		2	1		

TACO BELL

	Complete Protein Subgroup 2	Grain	Fat	Veg.	Fruit
Bean Burrito with Green or Red Sauce		3 1/2	2	1	
Beef Burrito with Green or Red Sauce	2	2	1	1	
Burrito Supreme with Green or Red Sauce	1	3	3		
Cinnamon Crispas		2	3		
Enchiritos with Green or Red Sauce	2	2	2		
Chicken Fajita	1	1	1	1	
Steak Fajita	1	1	1	1	
Meximelt	1	1	2	1	
Mexican Pizza	2	2 1/2	5	1	
Nachos		2 1/2	4		
Nachos Bellgrande	1	4	6		
Pintos and Cheese with Green or Red Sauce	1	1			
Chicken Taco	1	1	1		
Soft Taco	1	1	1	1	
Taco	1	1	1		
Taco Bellgrande	2	1	3		
Taco Light	2	1	4		
Tostada with Green or Red Sauce		1 1/2	2	1	
Ranch Dressing			5		
Salsa			1		
Sour Cream			1		

TACO JOHN'S
Burritos

	Complete Protein Subgroup 2	Grain	Fat	Veg.	Fruit
Bean Burrito	1	2		1	
Beef Burrito	2	2	2		
Combination Burrito	1	2	1		
Smothered Burrito with Texas Chili	2	3	3		
Super Burrito	1	3	2	1	

Chimichangas

	Complete Protein Subgroup 2	Grain	Fat	Veg.	Fruit
Chimichanga	1	4	3	1	
Chimichanga with Chicken	3	3	1	1	
Enchilada	2	2	2		

	Complete Protein Subgroup 2	Grain	Fat	Veg.	Fruit
Tacos					
Super Taco Bravo	1	3	3		
Taco	1	1	2		
Taco Brava	1	3	2		
Taco with Chicken	2	1			
Tostada	1	1	2		
Other Items					
Apple Grande		1	2		2
Mexican Rice		4	2		
Nachos		3	4		
Potato Ole Large		4	1		2
Refried Beans		5	1	1	
Super Nachos	2	4	5		
Texas Chili	2	2	2	1	

Food Group: Alcoholic Beverages

Current health guidelines advise that if you do drink alcoholic beverages, do so in moderation such as one to two standard-size drinks in a day. It is recommended that women refrain from drinking alcohol during pregnancy. If abstinence from alcohol is necessary for your recovery, avoid use of any alcoholic beverages including those listed below.

BEVERAGE	Grain	Fat	Fruit
Beer			
Extra Light, 12 oz.		2	
Light, 12 oz.	1	2	
Regular, 12 oz.	1	2	
Gin, 86 proof, 1 1/2 oz.		2	
Rum, 86 proof, 1 1/2 oz.		2	
Scotch, 86 proof, 1 1/2 oz.		2	
Vodka, 86 proof, 1 1/2 oz.		2	
Whiskey, 86 proof, 1 1/2 oz.		2	
Wine			
Champagne, 4 oz.		2	
Dry, white, 4 oz.		2	
Light, 4 oz.		1	
Port, 2 oz.	1/2	1	
Red, rose, 4 oz.		2	
Sherry, 2 oz.		1	
Sweet, 4 oz.	1/2	1	
Wine Cooler, 12 oz.		3	1 1/2

III. MISCELLANEOUS

A. Calcium Nutrition — Food Sources

Dairy products are the highest sources of calcium in the American food supply. Foods found in other groups provide lesser amounts of calcium. Recently, there has been an increased availability of calcium-fortified foods which can significantly improve calcium intake. The list below shows a comparison of the calcium content of foods *per unit* as found in your packet. To evaluate adequacy of your calcium intake, add up the total calcium content of foods written on each sample home menu and compare it with the recommended intake of calcium for your age in the Class Outline, "Calcium Nutrition — Osteoporosis and Eating Disorders."

HIGHEST CALCIUM SOURCES	Unit	Approximate mg of Calcium
Milk		
Whole, 2%, 1%, skim	1 cup	300
Chocolate, buttermilk	1 cup	285
Calci-Skim or other calcium-fortified milk	1 cup	400
Dried skim milk powder	1/3 cup	300
Cheese		
American, processed	1 oz.	175
Brick, Caraway, Cheddar, Colby, Edam, Monterey, Muenster	1 oz.	200
Cottage	1/4 cup	40
Ricotta, part skim	1/4 cup	170
Swiss	1 oz.	275
Cream cheese	1 oz.	25
Yogurt		
Flavored	1 cup	390
Fruit added	1 cup	345
Plain	1 cup	415

OTHER CALCIUM SOURCES		
Combination/International Foods		
Cheese pizza (14 – 16 oz.)	1/6	220
Chili with beans	1 cup	80
Cream soups made with milk	1 cup	180
Cream soups made with water	1 cup	30
Macaroni and Cheese	1 cup	360
Taco, beef and cheese	1	170
Complete Proteins		
Egg, large	1	30
Oysters, raw	1 cup	225
Salmon, canned, with bones	1 oz.	55
Sardines, canned, with bones	1 oz.	125
Shrimp, canned	1 oz.	35
Tofu processed with calcium sulfate	4 oz.	145
Desserts		
Cookies, chocolate chip, made with calcium-fortified flour	2	20
Cookies, chocolate chip, made with all-purpose flour (not calcium-fortified)	2	3
Ice cream	2/3 cup	120
Milkshake	1 cup	300
Pudding, custard	1/2 cup	140
Fat		
Cream cheese	1 Tbsp.	10
Fruit		
Orange juice or grapefruit juice, Citrus Hill calcium-fortified	1/2 cup	105
Rhubarb, cooked, sweetened	1/2 cup	100

	Unit	Approximate mg of Calcium
OTHER CALCIUM SOURCES (continued)		
Miscellaneous		
Blackstrap molasses	1 Tbsp.	135
Carnation Instant Breakfast Drink (1 packet + 1 cup milk)		610
Cornflakes, Total brand	³/₄ cup	120
Oatmeal, Total brand	¹/₂ cup	160
Pancakes, 4" diameter	2	115
Waffle, 7" diameter	1	180
Flour, Gold Medal brand calcium-fortified	¹/₂ cup	80
Vegetable		
Beet greens, cooked	¹/₂ cup	70
Broccoli	¹/₂ cup	70
Cabbage, bokchoy, cooked	¹/₂ cup	125
Collards, cooked	¹/₂ cup	150
Kale, cooked	¹/₂ cup	80
Mustard greens, cooked	¹/₂ cup	100
Turnip greens, cooked	¹/₂ cup	100

B. Definition of Terms

Calorie

A unit of measure to indicate the energy content of food. Calorie-carrying nutrients include carbohydrate, protein and fat.

Carbohydrate

The nutrient that is the major source of calories in a healthy meal plan. Carbohydrates are found in the various chemical forms of starches, sugars and fiber. Foods high in carbohydrate are listed in the grain, fruit, vegetable and sweets group.

Fat

The nutrient which supplies the most concentrated form of energy to the body. Foods containing fat provide these key nutrients: fat-soluble vitamins A, D, E, K and essential fatty acids. As a source of slower-release energy, fat aids in stabilizing the appetite between meals.

Fiber

The part of fruits, vegetables and whole grain products that are not digested by the body. Since various forms of fiber yield bulk to the diet, fiber aids in bowel regularity and in maintaining a healthy digestive system.

Meal Plan

A guide which shows the number of food units to eat from each food group every day.

Protein

A nutrient used to build and repair body tissue. Protein can also be used as an energy source by the body. Proteins are made up of 22 subunits called amino acids. Of these 22 amino acids, eight of them are termed "essential amino acids" since the adult cannot make them in adequate amounts to maintain health. Therefore, the body depends upon food sources to supply essential amino acids. In general, foods from animal sources (meat, egg and dairy products) provide liberal amounts of all amino acids and can be regarded as complete protein sources. Foods of plant origin (grains, fruits and vegetables) supply many amino acids, although not all essential amino acids in amounts needed by the body. These plant proteins, which can be viewed as incomplete proteins, enhance the body's use of essential amino acids.

Metabolism
   The chemical and physical processes of all cells in the body.

Minerals
   Substances needed by the body in small amounts. One mineral, calcium, plays a major role in bone health. Iron, another mineral, is part of the red blood cell which carries oxygen to all cells in the body.

Nutrition
   The intake and utilization of food to nourish the body.

Unit
   One serving of food from a food group.

Vitamins
   Substances "vital" for life but required in very small amounts. Vitamins do not contain calories; a major function in the body is involvement in chemical reactions that release energy from carbohydrates, proteins and fat.

C. Abbreviations

oz.	ounce
Tbsp.	tablespoon
tsp.	teaspoon

REFERENCES

1. U. S. Department of Agriculture, U.S. Department of Health and Human Services, *Nutrition and Your Health: Dietary Guidelines for Americans.* Washington, D. C., U. S. Government Printing Office, 3rd Ed., Home and Garden Bulletin No. 232, U. S. Government Printing Office, Washington, D. C., 1990.

2. Leonard, T., Mohs, M., Watson, R., The Effects of Caffeine on Various Body Systems — A Review, *J. Am. Diet. Assoc.,* 87, 1048, 1987.

3. The American Diabetes Association, Inc., The American Dietetic Association, *Exchange Lists for Meal Planning,* 1989.

4. Gordon, J., Marlatt, G. A., Eds., *Relapse Prevention: Maintenance Strategies in the Treatment of Addiction,* The Guilford Press, New York, 1985, 32-33.

CLASS OUTLINES

ACKNOWLEDGMENTS

I wish to acknowledge the expertise of Dr. David Abbott and other MeritCare Eating Disorders Program Staff who integrated the concepts of the three-dimensional model and the learning curve into the inpatient program design.

I. NUTRITION CLASS: THE DIETING ADDICTION

A. Introduction

Dieting is a strong driving force behind anorexia and bulimia. In order to recover, it is vital to stop the desire to lose weight. One is vulnerable to relapse (resuming eating disordered behavior) unless one accepts the concept of a healthy weight range.

B. Is Our Culture a Culprit?

1. Images of Thinness

Our society, through various methods of mass communication, sells the image of body thinness to the American public. Some examples of mass communication that convey exaggerated images of thinness include photographs of models on magazine covers, diet products/program advertisements, and television/movie stars.

2. Result

The result of this widespread bias of mass communication: Many Americans are unhappy with their bodies. Many people then try to diet to unhealthy, unrealistic weight goals. The negatives to this include poor self-esteem, wasted effort, undernutrition, and large sums of money spent on weight reduction products and programs.

3. How Common is Dieting?

How common is dieting in our country? Consider these reflections of unhappiness.

a. In a February, 1984 survey by *Glamour* magazine "Feeling Fat in a Thin Society," 75% of 33,000 women who responded thought of themselves as fat. Using medically accepted weight standards, only 25% of the women were considered to be overweight and *30% of the women were underweight*.[1] Of the underweight women, approximately half were still dieting through such health-threatening methods as crash diets, diet pills and laxatives.

b. It is estimated that 80% of American teenagers go on a diet before the age of 15.

c. From these "reflections of unhappiness," it appears that our society has gone too far in its obsession with thinness. *NOTE:* Being physically fit (good) is not the same as being excessively thin through chronic dieting.

4. Why Be Aware of Society's Pressures to be Ultra-thin?

a. One can actively choose not be "buy in" to the obsession of thinness.

b. One can improve self-esteem and become comfortable with a healthy weight range.

c. One can increase the desire to maintain healthy eating and exercise habits.

C. Set Point Theory of Weight Regulation

1. Theory

The set point theory offers an explanation of how the body "watches its weight." Two current versions of this theory are summarized.

a. **First version:** Each person has a unique *stable adult weight range* and *percentage of body fat*. This weight range is the point of balance in adult years where a person neither gains nor loses significant amounts of weight while eating according to appetite (not dieting) and adequately exercising. This weight range is also strongly influenced by genetics. The body is designed to actively defend its state of health; it cares about maintaining healthy weight and adequate fat stores. The body automatically keeps a stable weight range even though a person will have day-to-day minor variations in the amount of exercise done and calories consumed.

b. **Second version:** Each person has a genetically-influenced *calorie set point*. The body cares about how many calories are taken in. Furthermore, the body has many internal regulators which determine how calories are used: calories may be burned for immediate energy needs, stored as fat for future energy needs, or if consumed in excess, burned off in the form of heat. The goal of the calorie set point is to achieve a fairly even intake of calories each day and to use those calories in ways that aid in stabilizing a healthy weight range.

2. Research Supporting the Set Point Theory

a. **Dr. Ancel Keys.** University of Minnesota — Starvation Study. 1944[2]

Thirty-six healthy male volunteers were semi-starved for six months. They lost an average of 35 pounds or approximately 23% of their usual body weight. Various signs of starvation occurred during this six-month period. These signs of starvation (listed below) affected their feelings, thoughts and actions. These same signs are often seen in anorexia and in the combination of anorexia with bulimia.

- Obsession with thoughts of food and eating.

- Change in mood; increased irritability and depression.

- Decreased ability to concentrate and make decisions.

- Disturbance of sleep.

- Delayed movement of food passing through the stomach and intestinal tract resulting in bloating.

- Increased fatigue and apathy.

- Ongoing sensations of hunger.

After six months of dieting, the men were allowed to eat freely. The following observations were made.

- In the first week, the men gorged on 7,000 to 10,000 calories per day. Even on these high caloric intakes, some men still complained of hunger.

- After the first week, eating leveled off to 3,200 to 4,500 calories per day.

- When the men had gained enough to reach their usual (pre-experiment) weight, the hunger faded and the gorging stopped.

b. **Ethan Sims.** Vermont State Prison — Overfeeding Study. 1964[2]

Male volunteers ate two to three times more than their usual caloric intake. As expected, the men gained weight. However, it was *very difficult* for these men to gain weight even on such high levels of intake as 7,000 calories per day and with decreased activity. Once the men stopped overeating, all but two men rapidly lost weight until they were within 3 to 5 pounds of their usual (pre-experiment) weight.

Moral to These Studies

The body takes an active role in seeking out its individual, genetically-influenced set point. Efforts to force weight below the set point (dieting) are, at best, ineffective and temporary for most people.

D. Dieting: The Yo-Yo Trap

Many people go on and off reducing diets, as shown by the "reflections of unhappiness" discussed earlier. Research shows that there may be long-term health risks involved with repeated dieting attempts. For some people, their body's internal weight regulatory abilities (set point) can become distorted with yo-yo dieting. (Sections A and B that follow will explain how this distortion can occur.)

When a person goes on a diet and begins to lose weight, the body goes on the defensive. The body interprets dieting as a life-threatening occurrence (famine) and will work to preserve its own reserves of energy (fat and muscle tissue). These changes happen in response to dieting:

1. A Drop in Basal Metabolic Rate (BMR)

BMR = calories burned by the body for vital functions in the resting state (such as calories needed for breathing and for maintaining body temperature). Of a person's total calorie requirements, BMR accounts for 60 to 70% of this amount. In response to dieting, the BMR can begin dropping within 24 hours and continues to decline up to 20% in two weeks. In this way, the body begins to protect its own energy reserves and the dieter discovers that losing weight becomes more difficult — even on a lowered caloric intake.

2. Changes in Body Composition

The body, interpreting dieting as a life-threatening famine, chooses to minimize the amount of fat tissue being burned; fat tissue is held in reserve in case the "famine" lasts for a long time. The body, needing calories to fuel vital process (BMR), will then choose to burn both muscle and fat tissue (instead of just fat tissue). This leads to an undesirable loss of lean body tissue (muscle). When a person attempts to lose weight by dieting alone, a proportion of approximately 75% of calories burned comes from fat tissue and 25% of calories comes from lean body tissue. (This is a relatively high percentage of lean body tissue being burned for fuel.) For the dieter, this is a negative result. Loss of lean body tissue makes further weight loss more difficult because this type of tissue is metabolically very active; this tissue burns a significant amount of calories even when the body is at rest. In contrast, fat tissue is metabolically very sluggish; very few calories are burned by this tissue. The end result: Basal metabolic rate will decrease when lean body tissue is lost, making further weight loss more difficult.

When dieting is stopped, weight lost as muscle is often regained as fat. Over repeated on-and-off periods of dieting, the body may increase its proportion of fat tissue to lean body tissue. This in turn, may distort the body's set point and increase the percentage of fat tissue that the body wants to carry.

E. Metabolic Alterations with Eating Disorders

1. Anorexia Nervosa

Research has shown that at least through two or more months after reaching the healthy weight range, anorectic individuals require 30% to 50% more calories to maintain their healthy weight range than bulimic anorectics.[3] This is attributed to the fact that weight-restored anorectics burn calories faster than bulimic anorectics. Eventually (over several months) the basal metabolic rate will most likely decrease to normal; the body will not require a higher caloric intake to maintain the healthy body weight range. *Of interest:* Healthy weight gain for the recovering anorectic is a result of *both* restored muscle tissue and fat tissue. The weight gain is not all fat tissue, as is frequently thought by individuals with eating disorders.

2. Bulimia Nervosa

Studies indicate that the basal metabolic rate of bulimic individuals is reduced.[4] As a result, the body is inclined to store more calories consumed as fat tissue.

3. Metabolic Rates

A small number of available studies indicate that the metabolic rates of both anorectic and bulimic individuals can gradually return to normal following resumption of healthy eating habits.[3,5] However, the normalization of metabolic rate may occur over a period of months.

F. Is Weight Loss Desirable for Anyone?

For some adults, weight loss may be appropriate for health. Obesity (excessive stores of fat tissue) is one of several risk factors associated with heart disease, high blood pressure and diabetes.

Weight loss is not appropriate for a person with an eating disorder for whom the addiction to dieting must be broken. If an individual has become significantly overweight as a result of bulimia, any attempt at weight loss needs to be postponed until the active eating disorder has been resolved for some time.

Prolonged dieting during adolescence may result in an undesirable slowing of growth. A study of 19 overweight children showed that there was a decline in their rate of growth in height when following a mild calorie-restricted diet for weight loss.[6] Could this result in permanent stunting? The answer is not yet clear, but teenagers who have a long history of dieting should consider this possibility. Eating adequately during the growth years (up to 18 years for women, 21 years for men) will ensure that a person will reach full potential for height.

G. When Appropriate, How is Weight Loss Best Achieved?

For obese individuals who are medically at risk, a weight loss program ideally preserves health and lean body tissue. A good exercise program (30 minutes of aerobic exercise three to five times per week) and healthy eating habits (including a moderate intake of fats and desserts) will result in weight loss from the burning of predominantly fat tissue (instead of fat and muscle tissue).

Developing adequate exercise and healthy eating habits may allow the body to reduce the percentage of body fat it wants to carry. In this way, the body may adjust its set point to a lower (healthy) percentage of fat tissue.

H. Fad Diets — Common Clues

- Become Very Popular in a Short Time

- Sound Easy

- Promote a Specific Food or Food Group While Other Food Groups are Reduced or Avoided

- Distort Basic Nutrition Principles

I. Laxatives, Diet Pills and Diuretics: Playing With Fire

In order to lose weight, some individuals may turn to these over-the-counter products. These methods are not only ineffective in the long run, but may have dangerous side effects.

1. Laxatives

Laxative abuse is becoming more common. Individuals with eating disorders are most apt to use the stimulant-type laxatives. When taken in large amounts, the result is a watery diarrhea in which water and important minerals are lost. However, calories from foods eaten are not eliminated from the body by laxative use; almost all calories continue to be absorbed by the body. Studies have shown that even with extremely dangerous dosages of laxatives, only a small amount of calories (less than 12% of calories consumed) will be eliminated from the body. This is too high a price to pay!

2. Diet Pills

The key ingredient in diet pills is phenylpropanolamine (PPA). This chemical is similar to amphetamine. PPA is thought to reduce appetite, although its long-term effectiveness for weight control is considered to be minimal. After two to three weeks of taking products containing PPA, the effect of reducing appetite is lost unless the dosage is increased to dangerous levels. Undesirable side effects include anxiety, agitation, dizziness and high blood pressure. The Food and Drug Administration is currently reviewing the safety and effectiveness of PPA and is also likely to ban over 100 ingredients found in nonprescription diet pills due to their ineffectiveness.[7]

3. Diuretics

Diuretics cause temporary weight loss through increased loss of water as urine. This can lead to serious medical problems such as dehydration and loss of vital minerals which regulate many body functions.

J. Conclusion

Our society's bias for being ultra-thin is unrealistic for most adults. We don't have to "buy in" to these unrealistic and unhealthy images of the ultra-thin body.

Chronic and yo-yo dieting can have many negative long-term health consequences, particularly in its addictive forms of anorexia and bulimia. Some consequences include interference with growth, malnutrition leading to osteoporosis (thinning of bones), anemia, and perhaps long-term disturbance in the body's ability to self-regulate healthy weight.

Bulimia is an excellent way to gain weight. Many individuals with bulimia have gained weight significantly above their predisorder body weight. In the early months of recovery, *intentional weight loss* for these individuals is not desirable; the primary goal during this time is to relearn healthy eating habits. Therefore, the calorie level of the home meal plan will not be geared to initial weight loss. However, once the body is receiving a healthy intake of food (the home meal plan), the body's set point may operate in such a way as to lean gradually to an individual's predisorder healthy weight range.

A healthy lifestyle will enable the body to self-regulate its weight (set point). If one is healthy and fit, whatever size one is — is fine.

II. NUTRITION KNOW-HOW: INTRODUCTION TO MEAL PLANNING

A. Good Nutrition: A Definition

In 1990, nine major U.S. health organizations reached agreement on a current definition of healthy eating for Americans.

Their general recommendations are published in two reports, the "Healthy American Diet" and "Dietary Guidelines for Americans."[1, 2] These recommendations, listed below, apply to all healthy Americans over the age of two years:

1. Eat a variety of foods.

2. Maintain healthy weight.

3. Reduce consumption of dietary fat to 30% or less of the total caloric intake. Of total fat consumption, reduce intake of saturated fats and cholesterol.

4. Increase consumption of complex carbohydrates and dietary fiber with grain products, fruits and vegetables.

5. Use sugar and salt in moderation.

6. Drink alcoholic beverages in moderation, if at all.

B. Carbohydrate, Protein and Fat

The meal plan translates these recommendations into healthy food choices by means of the energy nutrients: carbohydrate, protein and fat.

1. Carbohydrate

a. Carbohydrate-rich foods include starchy foods (breads, cereals, potatoes, pasta) and foods with sugar (fruit, milk, desserts and table sugar).

b. The major function of carbohydrates is to supply a steady energy supply to the trillions of cells in the body.

2. Protein

a. Foods supplying high-quality protein include meat, eggs and many dairy products. Proteins of a lesser quality and concentration are found in gains, nuts, legumes and other plant sources.

b. Protein's major functions include building and repairing body tissues and maintaining an effective immune system with which to resist various illnesses. Proteins from foods which are not used for these vital functions are either used for energy or converted to fat tissue.

3. Fat

a. Common food sources of fat include margarine, butter, oils, meat, many dairy products and many desserts.

b. Dietary fat carries fat-soluble vitamins A, D E and K and supplies essential fatty acids to body cells.

c. Fat from foods is helpful in stabilizing appetite between meals because a relatively long period of time (approximately 4 hours) is needed to fully digest and absorb fat after being eaten. This prolonged action reduces "hunger pangs" between meals and may reduce the urge to binge.

d. Of the three energy nutrients, dietary fat is the most concentrated form of energy for the body. The body converts a certain amount of *dietary carbohydrate, protein* and *fat* into body fat reserves. Body fat reserves are the primary source of fuel used for prolonged exercise; fat reserves burned for energy provide "staying power". Body fat is the primary, most calorie-dense energy reserve in the body. Humans would be significantly larger if the primary energy reserve depended upon carbohydrates stored in the body.

e. Body fat serves as insulation, preventing excessive loss of body heat.

Table 1.
Comparison of Healthy Eating Recommendations and Actual Eating Practices

	CARBOHYDRATE		PROTEIN		FAT
Recommended ranges of intake	50–60% of total calories		13–20% of total calories		30% or less of total calories
Typical American eating patterns	35–40% of total calories		15–20% of total calories		40–50% of total

Meal Plan Groups	Complex	Simple	High Quality	Low Quality	Unsaturated/ Saturated
	Grain Veg group	Fruit group Sweets group Dessert group Milk group	Complete protein group Milk group	Grain group Veg group Fruit group	Complete protein group Fat group Dessert group

f. Body fat surrounds vital organs such as the heart, liver, kidneys and brain, acting as a shock absorber against injury.

C. Recommended Amounts of Carbohydrates, Protein and Fat

(Based upon an intake of 1,600 or more calories per day for an adult)

See Table 1, Comparison of Healthy Eating Recommendations and Actual Eating Practices

D. The Body's Energy Needs

The body runs 24 hours a day; body cells must have a continuous supply of energy in order to survive.

Calories consumed are either used for immediate energy needs, converted into short-term carbohydrate energy reserves (glycogen) or converted to the largest energy reserve (body fat).

Major Routes of Energy Usage

1. Basal metabolic needs: Calories are burned -around the clock- for functions even while the body is at rest. Such functions include breathing, heart muscle activity and maintenance of adequate body temperature.

2. Specific dynamic action: Calories are needed to fuel the additional processes of eating, digesting and absorbing foods.

3. Calories are burned for physical activity.

4. When excessive calories are consumed, the body may increase body heat production beyond normal levels in order to "burn off" unneeded calories. This may be one method the body uses to stabilize body weight/amount of fat tissue within the body's genetically-influenced "comfort zone" — the body's set point.

E. Scheduling of Meals

1. Routine mealtimes (a minimum of three meals per day at well-spaced intervals) is important in reestablishing normal appetite.

2. When food intake is spread throughout the day, more calories are used for digestion (thermic effect of food).

3. Individuals who skip breakfast may have metabolic rates 4% to 5% below normal.[3]

4. Spacing of meals allows dietary fat to work in reducing "hunger pangs" after eating. Overwhelming hunger is a risk situation for binge-eating.

5. On a three-meals-per-day eating schedule, the body simultaneously refills both carbohydrate energy reserves (glycogen) and body fat reserves. However, when a person skips meals, leading to periods of fasting, the body may overshoot the refilling of fat energy reserves when eating finally does occur. Over time, skipping meals may lead to increased body fat stores.

6. Large, infrequent meals, such as binge-eating, can result in very high levels of sugar from digested foods in the blood. This high blood sugar level may overstimulate the release of a hormone, insulin. Excessive amounts of insulin may rapidly drop the amount of sugar in the blood to very low levels, leading to the sensations of dizziness, fatigue and hunger.

F. Good Nutrition — Summary Statement

Healthy eating = a variety of foods + any one food or food group in moderation + routine mealtimes

G. Restaurant Eating Tips

Do not skip or shortchange any meal during the day when eating out. When preplanning the total daily intake of food, divide total food units somewhat evenly among the meals so that the appetite will stay on track. An individual can then look forward to feeling comfortably full after eating the restaurant meal.

If possible, eat at the same restaurants in order to become familiar with the types and amount of foods that are offered.

The meal planning system includes a restaurant section which lists specific food group units for products of some chain restaurants.

Complete proteins — estimating portion size

1. Visually compare the cooked meat entree with the palm of the hand. (A serving of meat that resembles the size of a woman's palm is approximately 3 ounces; for a man's palm, the meat would be approximately 4 ounces.) Alternatively, a serving of cooked meat resembling the size of a full deck of cards equals approximately 3 ounces.

2. The restaurant may offer reduced entree portions under the "for the lighter appetite" section, or the "senior citizens" section. In addition, some restaurants may designate moderate meat servings with a red heart or other symbol of the restaurant is participating in a "Heart Health" consumer education program.

3. It may be helpful to remember that the meal plan allows for the eating of up to three

additional food units beyond the plan on a given day. Therefore, additional units of complete protein may be chosen on this occasion.

Vegetable options: A tossed salad from the salad bar can represent one vegetable unit. If a vegetable choice is not available, an individual may choose to shorten the meal plan by one vegetable unit on that day or include the vegetable choices at another meal.

Fruit options: The salad bar may offer fresh fruit or a small order of juice may be available. Planning all fruit units in at other meals and snacks on that day is another option.

Fat units: If a dinner salad is served at the table, ask for the dressing on the side. The amount of dressing used can then be controlled.

Share a restaurant dessert with a companion; this "extra" may be enjoyed above planned meal units.

An eventual goal to discuss with the outpatient dietitian or counselor concerns the desire to eat a spontaneous, unplanned meal out. A helpful thought: One unplanned meal eaten each week represents only one out of 21 meals eaten per week! The set point theory allows for an occasional unplanned restaurant meal without experiencing significant weight changes.

III. CALCIUM NUTRITION: OSTEOPOROSIS AND EATING DISORDERS

A. Introduction

What is osteoporosis? This disease occurs as a result of gradual loss of structural bone minerals, especially calcium. Bones become weakened, brittle and potentially breakable. Body sites most commonly at risk for fracture are the hip and the spinal column.

Who is at risk? Middle-aged and older women (following menopause) and young women with chronic eating disorders are at highest risk for developing osteoporosis.

B. Bone Physiology

Bone is made up primarily of two types of tissue: (1) cortical (hard outer shell) and (2) trabecular (honeycomb-like inner support tissue).

Bone is active tissue. Bone is constantly being remodeled between the opposing action of the bone-*building* cells (osteo*b*lasts) and the bone-*crushing* cells (osteo*c*lasts).

From the years of adolescence to the mid-30's, the bone-building osteo*b*lasts work more than the bone-crushing osteo*c*lasts so the overall positive result is that calcium is being deposited in bone. Peak bone mass is achieved by the mid-30's. In later years, the osteo*b*lasts begin to decline while the osteo*c*lasts remain active. The overall result is that calcium is being removed from bone, especially the trabecular bone.

If an abnormally large amount of calcium is removed from bone, osteoporosis may occur.

C. What Causes Bone to Lose More Calcium Than It Should? (Risk factors for osteoporosis)

1. *Women* are at higher risk for developing osteoporosis than men since most women have smaller bones (a smaller calcium reserve).

2. A *family history of osteoporosis* which is often associated with small body frame (a smaller calcium reserve).

3. A female hormone, estrogen, better enables the bones to absorb calcium. In the years when estrogen levels are high (between adolescence and menopause), bone building is enhanced. *Following menopause*, estrogen is no longer produced, resulting in loss of calcium from bone.

4. Women who *smoke* experience menopause on average one to two years earlier than nonsmoking women. Therefore, women smokers prematurely lose the bone-building effects of estrogen.

5. *Exercise extremes* can upset the bone-building process. Excessive exercise can be harmful by decreasing estrogen levels to the point where menstruation does not occur. A decline in estrogen leads to bone loss in women. Very low levels of exercise also impair bone building. Adequate exercise is very important in maintaining well-mineralized bone. The most beneficial type of exercise places healthy stress on weight-bearing bones such as walking, cycling, jogging, tennis and aerobics. The optimal amount for bone building is approximately 30 minutes, four to five times per week. (This amount of exercise is also consistent with recommendations for heart health and for moderating appetite.)

6. An excessively *thin* person does not benefit from the bone-building effect of exercise as much as a person of average weight.

7. *Inadequate intake* of two key nutrients, *calcium* and *vitamin D*, will result in decreased bone building.

D. Is Osteoporosis Common in People with Eating Disorders?

1. In one study, 20 women ranging in age from 14 to 30 with chronic anorexia nervosa/loss of menstrual cycles were assessed for bone health. Fifteen of the 20 women had significant loss of minerals from their bones.[1]

2. In one study of 22 anorectic women, 77% had decreased bone density to the extent to place them at mild risk for fracture.[1]

3. Bone mineral density of eight bulimic women were compared to ten women without an eating disorder. Although all of the women consumed adequate amounts of calcium, bone mineral density was lower in all of the bulimic women. From this study, it appears that the amount of bone lost is associated with frequency of purging behaviors and length of time that a person has been bulimic.[2]

4. Some women whose chronic anorectic behaviors began at an early age have shown a decline in height. This may be caused in part to a collapsed spinal column from loss of bone.[3]

E. Why Are Persons with Eating Disorders at Risk for Developing Osteoporosis?

1. *Low estrogen levels* as evidenced by absent or irregular menstrual cycles impair the body's absorption of calcium.

2. *Low body weight* of the anorectic individual decreases the beneficial effect of exercise.

3. *Restrictive eating* often results in low intakes of calcium and vitamin D, key bone-building nutrients.

4. Bulimia may lead to a *disturbance of the body's chemical acid/base balance,* thereby decreasing the absorption of calcium from food.

F. *Osteoporosis: Prevention*

The best way to prevent severe bone loss is to maximize the bone-building processes from the most critical years of adolescence through the mid-30's. This results in an optimal reserve of calcium in the bone for which some of the calcium will be removed in years following menopause.

A recent study has shown that adequate calcium nutrition and exercise levels throughout the *lifespan* are influential in preserving bone health.[4]

Can premature loss of bone from eating disorders be reversed with good nutrition? Results of studies are mixed. In one study, 20 women who were anorectic for six years or more had significantly decreased bone density. For these women, bone density improved with increased weight and was normal in patients who had recovered from their eating disorder.[5]

G. Healthy Eating Habits for Bone Health

An adequate caloric intake is necessary to maintain a healthy weight range. A healthy weight range (1) restores adequate estrogen levels which enhance bone building and (2) healthy body weight stimulates bone building from moderate amounts of exercise.

Healthy food choices with a focus on calcium-rich foods enhance bone building in years before menopause and minimize bone loss in years following menopause.

1. The amount of calcium recommended to meet nutritional needs varies as shown below.[6]

Group	Age	Recommended Dietary Allowance for Calcium
Children	1-10	800 milligrams (mg)
Teenagers/Young Adults	11-24	1,200 mg
Men and Women	25-50	800 mg
Women	51+	1,200 mg
Men	51+	800 mg

2. Studies of actual food intake show that many women obtain only 400 to 500 milligrams of calcium from usual food choices. Inadequate intake of calcium may be caused by dislike of dairy products which are calcium-rich foods, frequent consumption of low

calcium beverages such as pop, coffee and tea in place of milk, and lactose intolerance (a more common type of milk intolerance).

3. Vitamin D is vital for the absorption of calcium in the body. Vitamin D is produced by the body when skin is exposed to sunlight. Certain foods also supply vitamin D such as fortified milk, eggs and fish.

4. Whenever possible, a home meal plan will include two or more servings from the milk group. If previous calcium intake has not met the recommended level of calcium for one's age, the best approach is to boost one's daily selection of calcium-rich foods. (See pages 56 and 57, Calcium Nutrition-Food Sources.) If unable to do so because of a strong dislike for dairy products or allergy to dairy products, a calcium or calcium-vitamin D supplement may be beneficial. Before taking a calcium supplement, check with your doctor.

5. Some people may experience discomfort (bloating, diarrhea) when consuming dairy products due to the inability to fully digest lactose, a sugar naturally found in milk. These people may be able to tolerate acidophilus-treated milk, live culture yogurt and cheese.[7]

6. In addition to calcium and vitamin D, other nutrients such as protein and phosphorus are vital for bone health. Therefore, an adequate intake of a variety of foods (the home meal plan) is the best way to obtain all nutrients required for maintenance of healthy bones.α

IV. PERSPECTIVES IN RECOVERY

A. Introduction

Two broad goals exist in recovery from an eating disorder: restoring physical health and preventing relapse (preventing the return of the eating disorder).

Section II offers a perspective on nutrition and its role in restoring health. Sections III and IV outline two powerful ideas that can strengthen one's ability to prevent relapse: the three-dimensional model of human experience and the learning curve.

B. How Important Is Good Nutrition to Health?

1. Health can be defined as a balance between key components of mental and physical well-being. Figure 1. Components of Health).

2. Mental and emotional health are dependent upon a solid foundation of physical health. Therefore, restoring physical health becomes the first focus in recovery.

3. Taking care of one's physical health is an expression of positive self-esteem.

4. If one or more components of health (shown in the diagram) is lacking or inadequate, other components can suffer. Some examples:

   • Low intake of food can upset the sleep cycle.

   • Low intake of food can impair athletic performance.

   • Low intake of food can lessen the ability to mentally concentrate and make decisions.

   • Low intake of food can cause irritability and mood swings.

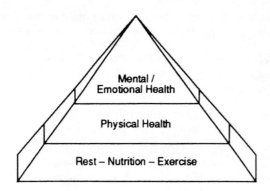

FIGURE 1. Components of health.

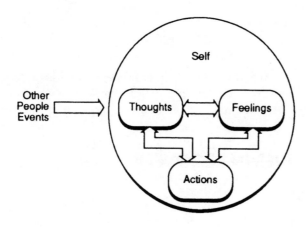

FIGURE 2. The 3-D model.

C. Three-Dimensional Model: How We Experience Life

We interpret and respond to people and events through three dimensions: our thoughts, our feelings and our actions.

Thoughts, feelings and actions interact and influence each other, most often without our awareness. Figure 2. The 3-D Model

Thoughts, feelings and actions are directed toward personal goals. This allows us to organize, and adjust our ongoing efforts toward achieving those goals. (Figure 3. The 3-D Model).

a.. **Thoughts** —In a healthy state, effective thought processes include problem-solving skills, decision-making abilities, priority setting, flexibility and positive thinking skills that enable a person to deal with stress.

b. **Feelings** — Our feelings are created from our thoughts; we are the author of our feelings. Other people or events do not produce one's feelings. In a healthy state, predominant feelings include happiness, positive self-esteem, and self confidence.

c. **Actions** — In a healthy state, our outward actions express and reinforce our inner thoughts and feelings. As an example, a person with positive self-esteem sets priorities and actions that will ultimately lead to achieving a goal. One of the basic priorities is to

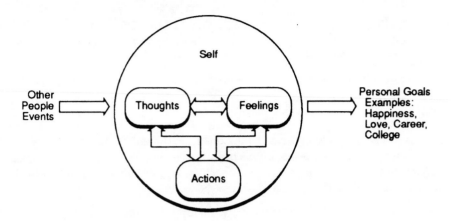

FIGURE 3. The 3-D model.

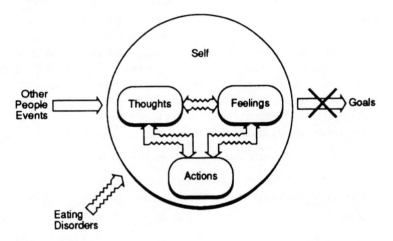

FIGURE 4. The 3-D model.

maintain physical health by taking time out for healthy eating, adequate exercise and sufficient rest.

2. Unhealthy State

The presence of an eating disorder can block/distort the constructive, goal-directed interactions of a person's thoughts, feelings, and actions. When this occurs, progress toward goals becomes impaired or blocked. (Figure 4. The 3-D Model).

a. **Thoughts** — An eating disorder frequently interrupts effective thought processes. Unproductive, inflexible thought processes occur.

- *Black-and-white thinking:* Food is judged to be either "good or bad," "safe or forbidden," leading to restrictive or unbalanced eating actions.

- *Catastrophizing:* A person with an eating disorder becomes overly fearful of future events; predictions are negative and are magnified. For example, "If I eat a cookie, I will gain 2 pounds and will fail my diet."

- *Perfectionism:* A person is very fearful of taking risks and of making mistakes. With this mindset, a person will establish unrealistic expectations. This becomes a set up for failure and low self-esteem.

In recovery, unhealthy thought processes of the person with an eating disorder are identified. Then, healthy thought processes are relearned through coaching and repetition.

b. **Feelings** — For the person with an eating disorder, unhealthy thought processes often lead to feelings of low self-esteem, anxiety and loneliness. *In recovery,* a person becomes aware of these self-made feelings and is able to gradually substitute healthy feelings as a response to healthy thoughts and actions.

c. **Actions** — In the initial stages of recovery, therapy is focused on changing unhealthy actions. (Actions are the easiest of the three dimensions to change.)

The meal plan is the tool to relearn healthy eating habits. The meal plan defines quality and quantity of foods to be eaten. In this way, foods are no longer labeled as "good or bad"; foods from all food groups can fit in the home meal plan.

Other healthy actions aid in recovery. One important step in maintaining recovery is to identify high-risk situations/feelings/thoughts that may cause a return to the eating disorder. Examples of high-risk situations may be grocery shopping, eating former binge foods, looking in a mirror, and eating out. Once these high-risk situations/feelings/thoughts are identified, *alternative healthy actions* are used in response to defuse these potentially harmful high-risk areas when they arise.

Examples of alternative healthy actions include:

- Go for a walk or call a friend when the urge to binge or negative thinking persists.

- Go grocery shopping with a friend.

- Avoid high-risk binge foods early in recovery. When reintroducing former binge foods, purchase only a single portion, such as one ice cream cone or one cookie at a bakery.

- If certain fast food restaurants trigger the urge to binge, alter the route of travel in order to minimize the temptation.

A key question that an individual with an eating disorder needs to consider is: Has the eating disorder been helpful in achieving personal goals? Most often the eating disorder has disrupted the person's progress in achieving goals. Recognizing this reality may strengthen one's desire to recover.

D. Learning Curve (See Figure 5. The Learning Curve)

Recovery will require time and will most likely include short periods of setbacks (slips) as an individual encounters former high-risk situations, thoughts and feelings.

"Ups and downs" will occur; as time goes on and healthy eating/living becomes more automatic, there will be fewer "downs." Recovery will run a smoother course with time and commitment.[1, 2]

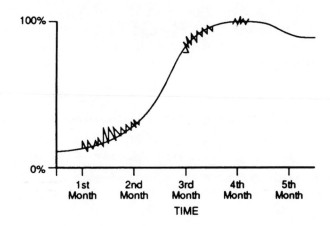

FIGURE 5. The learning curve.

REFERENCES

The Dieting Addiction

1. Feeling Fat in a Thin Society, *Glamour*, 198, Feb. 1984.

2. Bennett, W., and Gurin, J., *The Dieter's Dilemma*, Basic Book, Inc., New York, 1982, 11-19.

3. Ebert, M., George, T., Gwirtsman, H., Jimerson, D., Kaye, W., and Obarzanek, E., Calorie Intake Necessary for Weight Maintenance in Anorexia Nervosa: Nonbulimics Require Greater Caloric Intake than Bulimics, *Am. J. Clin. Nutr.*, 44, 435, 1986.

4. Ireton-Jones, C., and Sedlet, K., Energy Expenditure and the Abnormal Eating Pattern of a Bulimic: A Case Report, *J. Am. Assoc.*, 89, 74, 1989.

5. Ebert, M., George, T., Gwirtsman, H., Kaye, W., and Petersen, R., Caloric Consumption and Activity Levels After Weight Recovery in Anorexia Nervosa: A Prolonged Delay in Normalization, *Int. J. Eating Disorders*, 5:No. 3, 503, 1986.

6. Dietz, W., and Hartung, R., Changes in Height Velocity of Obese Preadolescents During Weight Reduction, *Am. J. Dis. Child*, 139, 705, 1985.

7. Food and Drug Administration, *Nonprescription Diet Drugs*, News Release, P90-50, 1990.

Nutrition Know-How: Introduction to Meal Planning

1. American Heart Association, *The Healthy American Diet*, 1990.

2. U. S. Department of Agriculture, U. S. Department of Health and Human Services, *Nutrition and Your Health: Dietary Guidelines for Americans*, 3rd Ed., Home and Garden Bulletin No. 232, U. S. Government Printing Office, Washington, D. C., 1990.

3. Hackman, E., Jump-Start Your Day, *Am. Health*, 2, 118, 1989.

Calcium Nutrition: Osteoporosis and Eating Disorders

1. Raymond, C., Long-term Sequelae Pondered in Anorexia Nervosa, *J. Am. M. Assoc.*, 257, 3324, 1987.

2. Brewer, M., Hegsted, M., Howat, P., Mills, G., and Varner, L., The Effect of Bulimia Upon Diet, Body Fat, Bone Density and Blood Components, *J. Am. Diet. Assoc.*, 89, 929, 1989.

3. Brotman, A., and Stern, T., Osteoporosis and Pathologic Fractures in Anorexia Nervosa, *Am. J. Psychiatry*, 142:4, 495, 1985.

4. Dalle, G., Dawson-Hughes, B., Krall, E., Sadowski, L., Sahyoun, J., and Tannerbaum, S., A Controlled Trial of the Effect of Calcium Supplementa-

tion on Bone Density in Postmenopausal Women, *N. Engl. J. Med.*, 323, 878, 1990.

5. Fogelman, I., Murby, B., Russell, G., and Treasure, J., Reversible Bone Loss in Anorexia Nervosa, *Br. Med. J.*, 295, 474, 1987.

6. Food and Nutrition Board, National Academy of Sciences — National Research Council, *Recommended Dietary Allowances*, National Academy Press, Washington, D. C., 1989.

Perspectives in Recovery

1. Garfinkel, P., and Garner, D., *Handbook of Psychotherapy for Anorexia and Bulimia*, The Guilford Press, New York, 1985, 554.

2. Gordon, J., and Marlatt, G. A. Eds., *Relapse Prevention: Maintenance Strategies in the Treatment of Addiction*, The Guilford Press, New York, 1985, 25.

INDEX

INDEX